Tensions and Barriers in
Improving Maternity Care

Tensions and Barriers in Improving Maternity Care

THE STORY OF A BIRTH CENTRE

RUTH DEERY
Reader in Midwifery
Centre for Health & Social Care Research
The University of Huddersfield

DEBORAH HUGHES
Community Midwifery Team Leader
Bradford Teaching Hospitals NHS Foundation Trust

and

MAVIS KIRKHAM
Emeritus Professor of Midwifery
Sheffield Hallam University

Foreword by

SHEILA KITZINGER

Radcliffe Publishing
Oxford • New York

Radcliffe Publishing Ltd
18 Marcham Road
Abingdon
Oxon OX14 1AA
United Kingdom

www.radcliffe-oxford.com
Electronic catalogue and worldwide online ordering facility.

British Library Cataloguing in Publication Data

A catalogue record for this book is available from the British Library.

ISBN-13: 978 184619 425 2

Typeset by Pindar NZ, Auckland, New Zealand
Printed and bound by Cadmus Communications, USA

Contents

Foreword

Here is a remarkably detailed analysis of the politics of a birth centre trapped in a medicalised system that threatened and rapidly destroyed it. It is a vivid example of how autonomous midwifery is undermined by an organisational structure in which management focuses exclusively on one model of care, namely midwifery training in obstetric emergencies and rescuing women from their inherently defective bodies, rather than safeguarding normal birth.

It tells of how midwives were pitted against each other, the failure to stimulate widespread support from the local community, and the use of already overworked community midwives to staff the birth centre. The centre restricted its opening hours to daytime only, and put severe limits on the time mothers and babies could stay there postpartum. It was not the birth centre that failed, but an authoritarian and bureaucratic hospital-based maternity system that was insensitive both to women's experiences there and to midwives' values and relationships.

This is an object lesson in how not to do it.

Sheila Kitzinger
April 2010

Sheila Kitzinger is a social anthropologist of birth, and her 24 books on pregnancy, childbirth and midwifery have been published around the world.

Preface

We have written this book because the story that it tells warrants a wide audience. The data that we collected from the midwives and others whom we interviewed were both more moving and more depressing than we had expected when we set out to inquire into why this birth centre had not been a success. To condense the narrative into the strictures of one or two academic papers would have meant that the full story would lose its place in the bigger world of maternity care. We also wrote this book because we know that there are many birth centres being established, and that both the literature and conferences tend to present the 'success stories' rather than the fuller picture, from which many equally valuable lessons can be learned.

However, this book is not just about one particular birth centre. Many of the issues and behaviours that we present here are echoed in other maternity services and midwifery experiences, and are replicated in situations where no birth centre exists. The maternity services and the experiences of all too many midwives working in them share many of the elements described here. Lack of leadership, support, vision and plain dealing is widespread, and as a result many midwives are thwarted from practising midwifery as they would wish. As a result, women are prevented from having the choices and services that they are entitled to expect from the National Health Service. We know that these problems are not unique to the UK. Our conversations with midwives from many countries highlight the fact that this is a very widespread problem, and demonstrate the tensions between bureaucracy and woman-centred care.

We see the purpose of this book as informing discussion and decision making around reconfigurations of maternity care, so that planning, communication, management and recruitment can be improved, and shared vision can be articulated and understood. It demonstrates the dangers of playing politics (with a small 'p') with a service that is so fundamentally important to the lives of women and local communities. We also hope that there will be more publications and presentations in the future that explore the 'dark side' of midwifery initiatives, so that a more realistic picture is presented of what it feels like to be a midwife in twenty-first-century Britain – the hopes and aspirations, the disappointments and hurts, the blood, sweat and tears, the vision and the commitment, the disillusionment and frustrations, and the pleasures and rewards.

New birth centres are opening every year, and older ones are closing. In the UK there are approximately 120 birth centres at the present time (about 90 in England, and the other 30 spread across Wales, Scotland and Northern Ireland). Further information can be found at www.babycentre. co.uk/pregnancy/labourandbirth/planningyourbabysbirth/birthcentre. The government advocates choice for women, and promotes birth centres as an option for low-risk women (Shribman, 2007). However, this policy ignores the problematic stories of many current and past birth centres. In the current economic climate, we are also anxious that sad tales of shelved or closed birth centres may become more rather than less common. It is in this context that we have decided to write the tale of this birth centre and its valiant but embattled midwives.

Ruth Deery, Deborah Hughes and Mavis Kirkham
April 2010

REFERENCE

Shribman S. *Making it Better: for mother and baby.* London: Department of Health; 2007.

About the authors

Ruth Deery is Reader in Midwifery at the University of Huddersfield. Over a career spanning 34 years she has worked continuously as a midwife and academic. She worked for many years on a large busy delivery suite, but now works in birth centres and community midwifery.

As an academic, her key interest at doctoral level was in applying sociological theory and action research methodology to the organisational culture of midwifery in the National Health Service in England. Since then her work has been mainly in the maternity services and women's health in the new NHS, with particular interests in organisational change, public policy, and emotions and care. Her research findings have been widely published in refereed journals.

Deborah Hughes is a community midwifery team leader in Bradford. Over 28 years as a midwife she has worked as a hospital and community midwife, an independent midwife, a researcher and a university teacher, in a Sure Start project, and in two birth centres. Her interests are midwife-led care and normal birth, and she has undertaken a number of research projects and written widely for the midwifery press. She lives in Yorkshire with her daughter and her dog, and her hobbies are walking, gardening and cookery.

Mavis Kirkham is Emeritus Professor of Midwifery at Sheffield Hallam University. She has worked continuously as a researcher and a clinical midwife for over 30 years. She would describe herself as a hybrid researcher, having worked in the disciplines of social anthropology, sociology, politics and history, using qualitative, observational and ethnographic methods as well as surveys and archive work. Her abiding research interest is in people's relationship with, and efforts to control, their work and its setting. Her clinical work is now mainly concerned with home births.

Approaching the end of a long career in midwifery, she is now interested in reflecting and writing on midwifery in its wider context. Her central professional concern is with normal birth, the conditions that foster it, and its enabling effects upon mothers, families and midwives. She has long been concerned with how birth stories are negotiated and adjusted, and the impact of these stories.

Authors' note

In order to protect all those involved, we agreed with senior management in the NHS trust concerned to anonymise the research site. This was done so that we would be able to explore in detail a process that has occurred in many places. It is relatively common to publish success stories, but stories of problems in maternity services are less common. We think that there is much to be learned from such stories, but as they can be painful for all involved, we wish to protect those individuals.

One problem with anonymising the site is that we cannot cite an earlier study which showed high levels of user satisfaction with the service provided there. We hope that we may be trusted in this regard, not least because so many other studies have shown high levels of satisfaction with birth centre services.

CHAPTER 1

Birth centres

BACKGROUND TO THE STUDY

Birth centres are defined and organised differently in different places, and some bear other names. Indeed the birth centre studied here has been organised in several different ways during its relatively short history. Hall (2003) describes 'free-standing low-risk maternity units' which are defined by their separation from a consultant maternity unit; other birth centres are sited alongside or within the same building as a consultant maternity unit. More importantly, the term 'birth centre' represents 'a set of values and beliefs about birth, without which it has little meaning' (Shallow, 2003, p. 12). This philosophy is 'centred on the concept of midwifery being at the heart of a social [rather than a medical] model of care' (Shallow, 2003, p. 13), in which midwives give skilled support and 'within which women can achieve normal, physiological birth' (Shallow, 2003, p. 13).

Such units, although described as a choice which should be available to women at low obstetric risk (Department of Health, 1993, 2004, 2005, 2007), are markedly different from the centralised, medicalised large maternity units, which operate on an industrial model and provide the setting in which the vast majority of babies are born. In 2007, the Department of Health restated its support of birth centres as a means of improving maternity care and offering choice to women (Shribman, 2007), and as a means of improving access to care for women from disadvantaged and vulnerable groups (Department of Health, 2004, 2007).

A number of studies have demonstrated that, when evaluated against obstetric outcomes of safety, births for low-risk women are at least as safe in birth centres as in hospitals (Kirkham, 2003; Walsh, 2007; Hatem *et al.*, 2008; Sandall *et al.*, 2009). There are two possible reasons for the good clinical outcomes associated with birth centres. First, birth may be safe for low-risk women because the gains of 'high-tech' settings are offset by the iatrogenic risks that they pose. Secondly, the very different philosophy and skills used by all involved in birth centres may make a positive difference. These factors, which result in safety, are probably impossible to separate.

As well as safe clinical outcomes, care in birth centres is linked with high levels of satisfaction. This is evident with regard to maternal satisfaction in a number of studies (Kirkham, 2003; Walsh, 2007; Hatem *et al.*, 2008). It is noteworthy that satisfaction is also reported by socially marginalised women from several cultures (Esposito, 1999). Fathers expressed satisfaction with the support and respect that they received in the birth centre in Stockholm (Waldenström, 1999), reflecting the focus of birth centre care upon the family rather than solely on the birth. It is interesting that the feeling of being 'treated with respect' is reported in these evaluations, particularly with regard to groups which often do not report such treatment (Esposito, 1999; Waldenström, 1999). Such perceptions of respect echo the emphasis that birth centre midwives place upon facilitating supportive relationships around birth. In enhancing the satisfaction of families, birth centre midwives are clearly doing something positive and empowering, and not just avoiding iatrogenesis. More work is needed to identify and describe what happens during birth centre care to give such positive outcomes, and such research will help the development of midwifery (Hughes and Deery, 2002).

Midwives also report satisfaction with working in birth centres (e.g. Saunders *et al.*, 2000; Kirkham, 2003), relishing the challenges offered by the difference from working in hospitals, and the greater responsibility involved.

Birth centres, under various names, have long been part of maternity care in the UK. They induce great loyalty in those who use them and work in them. Nevertheless, despite their clinical effectiveness and the satisfaction of their users and workers, there is considerable tension concerning the availability of this model of care, which deviates greatly from mainstream UK obstetrics.

BACKGROUND AND CONTEXT

Any change in maternity care has to be seen in the context of the wider situation in society, in the National Health Service (NHS), and in public services in general at the time of its introduction. In recent years, technical intervention in childbirth has increased greatly, with little improvement in clinical outcomes (NHS Institute for Innovation and Improvement, 2006). This reflects changing social attitudes to pain, choice and technology.

> . . . many of the social and cultural values, such as convenience, ease and control, that underpin Western society in the 21st century correlate with what intervention has to offer, which results in intervention being increasingly sought after and utilised. This milieu of intervention, which increasingly surrounds childbirth, is shown to be calling into question those things that have traditionally been at the heart of childbirth: the ability of the woman to birth and the clinical skills of the health professional. (McAra-Couper, 2007, p. ix)

The aims of a birth centre relate to values that were prevalent before such recent changes, and therefore create some tensions for all concerned. They may also be seen as a gauge that indicates current social changes in progress which are revaluing human relationships with regard to technology and medicine (Hunter *et al.*, 2008).

The birth centre studied here was set up at a time of frequent and continuing reorganisation of public services, together with policy priorities to run such services efficiently and economically. Although none of these pressures are new (Lipsky, 1980), the year-on-year requirements for economies and reorganisation have created mounting pressure on those providing services.

Within maternity care, service users and providers are aware of a growing tension between the rhetoric of public policy to provide women with choice, control and continuity of care, and the reality of staff shortages and increasing centralisation of services. Many midwives have responded to the mounting pressures upon them by reducing their working hours (Kirkham *et al.*, 2006) or by leaving midwifery (Ball *et al.*, 2002). Although the adjustment of midwifery staffing figures in the face of economic stringencies may cloak the shortage of midwives, a vicious circle has been created in which midwives experience frustration because they cannot practise as they wish. Midwives leaving the profession leads to increased work for those remaining, and the situation becomes ever more acute.

Centralisation of services has been a key feature of the organisation of maternity care in recent years. This economically led movement runs in uneasy counterpoint with the concurrent rhetoric of public policy concerning clients' choice. Many large cities now have one maternity unit with an annual birth rate far higher than anything in this country in the past or elsewhere in Europe at present. We are unaware of any research that demonstrates the long-term economic benefits of centralisation of services that are claimed when hospital closures are planned. However, centralisation does have various consequences, and can present opportunities for innovative service reconfiguration. Some highly successful birth centres have emerged as a result of the closure of maternity hospitals (e.g. Jones and Walker, 2003). Nevertheless, the pressures and fears generated by frequent, major service changes have led many NHS workers and service users to see the words 'reconfiguration', 'closure' and 'centralisation' as interchangeable. As Macfarlane (2008) has clearly pointed out, there are problems associated with larger units and reconfigurations and the potential for consequent detrimental effects on care. Furthermore, there has been no systematic analysis concerning the size of these units and the quality of the clinical care that they deliver (Macfarlane, 2008).

Another key factor in modern maternity care is the standardisation of services that has resulted from the proliferation of policies, protocols and clinical guidelines. Two major factors have fuelled the standardisation of practice. Initially this developed from efforts to provide clinical care based upon research evidence (Sackett *et al.*, 1996, 1997). Secondly, and more recently, standardisation has accelerated following the growing emphasis upon clinical governance in the NHS, especially in maternity care, where litigation is very costly. The requirements of the Clinical Negligence Scheme for Trusts (NHS Litigation Authority, 2009) link guidelines to costs, and add a further economic imperative to the many pressures to standardise care. In Chapter 9 we shall discuss the conceptualisation by Stronach *et al.* (2002) of professional identity as caught between such 'economies of performance' and 'ecologies of practice.'

The habits and vocabulary of proceduralisation, originally based upon research evidence, lead to expectations of standardised behaviour and a 'right way' for clinicians to act in any situation. This situation usually reflects the culture of the local service, and may pay little heed to individual women's circumstances, needs and expectations (Kirkham and Stapleton, 2001). Behaving in the 'right way' or becoming 'obedient technicians' (Deery and Hunter, 2010) gives midwives and obstetricians the security afforded by clinical governance, but can be seen as protecting the organisation rather than its users or clinicians. Such rule following is described by a colleague of ours as 'teflon-coated management', to which neither blame nor responsibility can adhere.

In a study of midwives returning to practice, and therefore able to make comparisons across time, it was found that returning midwives saw standardisation as improving the service for clients in some respects, but also as reducing opportunities for midwives to use their clinical judgement to tailor care to the needs of individual women. In a climate of fear of litigation and defensive practice, together with shortage of staff and pressure to get through the work, delivery of the standardised package of care is seen as a professional duty, and individualised care as being lost due to lack of time (Kirkham and Morgan, 2006; Bryson and Deery, 2009).

Hochschild described a 'professional' flight attendant as 'one who has completely accepted the rules of standardisation' (Hochschild, 1983, p. 103). 'By linking standardisation to honour and the suggestion of autonomy', and by identifying the work as 'professional', both flight attendants and midwives practise in a highly controlled manner. It is interesting that many aspects of the standardisation of practice originated from the aviation industry. Yet such Taylorist control (Torrington *et al.*, 2002) of the details of work within service organisations creates considerable moral dilemmas and occupational stress for midwives, especially within hospitals. It is also possible to envisage that the comprehensive protocolisation of clinical practice will interfere with professional progression 'from novice to expert' (Benner, 1984), because of the discouragement of intuitive caregiving (Drummond and Standish, 2007; Ilott and Cooke, 2007).

Expectation of standardisation makes it difficult for management and staff to envisage different ways of providing care, to innovate on a small scale or to create pilot schemes. Protocolisation of care is seen as superseding old ways. This is one reason why problems are encountered in maintaining home birth services in many areas, while prioritising the resource needs of a modern central delivery suite. Birth centres represent an aspect of maternity care that has a long history (such as the earlier general practitioner (GP) maternity homes), so their introduction may now be seen as a backward step or as a deviation from modern maternity care. Birth centres (and home birth) are difficult to tolerate when the 'right' way to give birth has been established as medicalised care in a consultant unit.

Midwives and their managers are increasingly aware of, and even more cynical about, changes in the language of policy that repackage previously negative concepts as positive. 'Reconfiguration' is a modern packaging of what were previously termed 'cuts and closures.' A shortage of, or reduction in, professional clinical staff is repackaged as 'skill mix.' Cuts in the number of antenatal and postnatal visits to women at home have been described as 'individualised care', although midwives find it difficult to increase the care of particularly needy women. Similarly, 'protocol-based care' (Malone and Fontenia, 2007; Ilott and Munroe, 2008) is positively packaged as evidence based and managing risk, but may not respond to the needs and wishes of individual women. We have heard such terminology referred to as 'menu midwifery.' This is not to say that any of these modern initiatives are without merit. However, the language in which they are presented, the intolerance of any alternatives (Jowett, 2009; Kirkham, 2009), and the identification of these initiatives with ongoing efforts to reduce costs all lead to cynicism among clinical midwives.

For midwifery and for low-risk birth, recent changes in the NHS have produced both losses and gains. Constant change and shortages of staff have wearied and demoralised midwives (Deery, 2005; Deery and Fisher, 2010). The gap between the rhetoric of choice and woman-centred care and the reality of centralised services in vast hospitals is striking. Yet clinical advances are made and reorganisation can present opportunities, one of which is studied here, together with the tensions of its context.

REFERENCES

Ball L, Curtis P, Kirkham M. *Why Do Midwives Leave?* London: Royal College of Midwives; 2002.

Benner P. *From Novice to Expert: excellence and power in clinical nursing practice.* Menlo Park, CA: Addison-Wesley; 1984.

Bryson V, Deery R. Public policy, 'men's time' and power: the work of midwives in the British National Health Service. In: *Women's Studies International Forum*, 2009. doi:org/10.1016/j.wsif.2009.11.004.

Deery R. An action research study exploring midwives' support needs and the effect of group clinical supervision. *Midwifery.* 2005; 21: 161–76.

Deery R, Fisher P. 'Switching and swapping faces': performativity and emotion in midwifery. *International Journal of Work, Organisation and Emotion.* 2010; 3: 270–86.

Deery R, Hunter B. Emotion work and relationships in midwifery: enhancing or challenging? In: M Kirkham (ed.) *The Midwife–Mother Relationship*, 2nd edn. Basingstoke: Palgrave Macmillan; 2010.

Department of Health. *Changing Childbirth. Part 1. Report of the Expert Maternity Group.* London: Department of Health; 1993.

Department of Health. *National Service Framework for Children, Young People and Maternity Services.* London: Department of Health; 2004.

Department of Health. *Creating a Patient-Led NHS.* London: Department of Health; 2005.

Department of Health. *Maternity Matters: choice, access and continuity of care in a safe service.* London: Department of Health; 2007.

Drummond J, Standish P. *The Philosophy of Nurse Education.* Basingstoke: Palgrave Macmillan; 2007.

Esposito NW. Marginalised women's comparisons of their hospital and free-standing birth centre experiences: a contrast of inner-city birthing systems. *Health Care for Women International.* 1999; **20:** 111–26.

Hall J. Free-standing maternity units in England. In: M Kirkham (ed.) *Birth Centres: a social model for maternity care.* Oxford: Books for Midwives; 2003. pp. 3–10.

Hatem M, Sandall J, Devane D *et al.* Midwife-led versus other models of care for childbearing women. *Cochrane Database of Systematic Reviews.* 2008; **4:** CD004667.

Hochschild AR. *The Managed Heart: commercialization of human feeling.* Berkeley, CA: University of California Press; 1983.

Hughes D, Deery R. Where's the midwifery in midwife-led care? *The Practising Midwife.* 2002; **5:** 18–19.

Hunter B, Berg M, Lundgren I *et al.* Relationships: the hidden threads in the tapestry of maternity care. *Midwifery.* 2008; **24:** 132–7.

Ilott I, Cooke J, Patterson M *et al. Standardising Care: it is shaping your practice?* Paper presented at the Community Practitioners and Health Visitors Association (CPHVA) Annual Professional Conference, 31 October – 2 November 2007, Torquay.

Ilott I, Munro J, Patterson M *et al. Clinical Guidelines: challenging midwives' autonomy and women's choice.* Paper presented at the International Confederation of Midwives (ICM) Triennial Congress 2008, 1–5 June 2008, Glasgow.

Jones O, Walker J. From concept to reality: developing a working model of a stand-alone birth centre. In: M Kirkham (ed.) *Birth Centres: a social model for maternity care.* Oxford: Books for Midwives; 2003. pp. 79–88.

Jowitt M. Save the Albany. *Midwifery Matters.* 2009; **123:** 2.

Kirkham M (ed.). *Birth Centres: a social model for maternity care.* Oxford: Books for Midwives; 2003.

Kirkham M. In fear of difference. *Midwifery Matters.* 2009; **123:** 7–9.

Kirkham M, Stapleton H (eds). *Informed Choice in Maternity Care: an evaluation of evidence-based leaflets*. York: NHS Centre for Reviews and Dissemination; 2001.

Kirkham M, Morgan RK. *Why Midwives Return and their Subsequent Experience*. London: Department of Health; 2006. www.nhsemployers.org and www.rcm.org (accessed 5 December 2009).

Kirkham M, Morgan RK, Davies C. *Why Midwives Stay*. London: Department of Health; 2006. www.nhsemployers.org and www.rcm.org (accessed 5 December 2009).

Lipsky M. *Street-Level Bureaucracy: dilemmas of the individual in public services*. New York: Russell Sage Foundation; 1980.

McAra-Couper J. *What is shaping the practice of health professionals and the understanding of the public in relation to increasing intervention in childbirth? A critical hermeneutic study*. PhD thesis. Auckland, New Zealand: Auckland University of Technology; 2007.

Macfarlane A. Reconfiguration of maternity units – what is the evidence? *Radical Statistics*. 2008; **96**: 77–86.

Malone JR, Fontenia M. *Protocol-Based Care*. London: National Coordinating Centre for NHS Service Delivery and Organisation R&D; 2007.

NHS Institute for Innovation and Improvement. *Delivering Quality and Value: focus on normal birth and reducing Caesarean section rates*. Coventry: NHS Institute for Innovation and Improvement; 2006.

NHS Litigation Authority. *Pilot Maternity Clinical Risk Management Standards*. London: NHS Litigation Authority; 2009.

Sackett DL, Rosenberg WMC, Gray JAM *et al*. Evidence-based medicine: what it is and what it isn't. *British Medical Journal*. 1996; **312**: 71–2.

Sackett DL, Richardson WS, Rosenberg WMC *et al*. *Evidence-Based Medicine*. London: Churchill Livingstone; 1997.

Sandall J, Hatem M, Devane D *et al*. Discussion of findings from a Cochrane Review of midwife-led versus other models of care for childbearing women: continuity, normality and safety. *Midwifery*. 2009; **25**: 8–13.

Saunders D, Boulton M, Chapple J *et al*. *Evaluation of the Edgware Birth Centre*. London: Barnet Health Authority; 2000.

Shallow H. The birth centre project. In: M Kirkham (ed.) *Birth Centres: a social model for maternity care*. Oxford: Books for Midwives; 2003. pp. 11–24.

Shribman S. *Making it Better: for mother and baby*. London: Department of Health; 2007.

Stronach I, Corbin B, McNamara O *et al*. Towards an uncertain politics of professionalism: teacher and nurse identities in flux. *Journal of Education Policy*. 2002; **17**: 109–38.

Torrington D, Hall L, Taylor S. *Human Resource Management*, 5th edn. Harlow: Pearson Education Limited; 2002.

Waldenström U. Effects of birth centre care on fathers' satisfaction with care, experience of the birth and adaptation to fatherhood. *Journal of Reproductive and Infant Psychology.* 1999; **17**: 357–68.

Walsh D. *Improving Maternity Services: small is beautiful – lessons from a birth centre.* Oxford: Radcliffe Publishing Ltd; 2007.

CHAPTER 2

The research story

This birth centre (hereafter referred to as the Birth Centre) was intended to be a homely, community-based, freestanding facility that would provide midwifery care 24 hours a day, seven days a week for local residents and other women who preferred a low-intervention approach to birth. Initially the Birth Centre was managed along these lines, staffed by midwives skilled in supporting women through normal birth, and providing individualised and family-centred care. However, in 2005, three years after the Birth Centre had opened, a crisis situation was reported to one of the researchers by the Head of Midwifery. We were told that the midwives were not promoting the Birth Centre facility and were resisting the potential to move clinical practice forward. What had previously been described as 'the jewel in the crown' was fast becoming 'a problem child.'

This research was therefore commissioned by the Head of Midwifery at the NHS trust where the Birth Centre was situated. The research was funded by small grants from the NHS trust and the University of Sheffield. Further funding was sought without success. Given the limited financing for the research, we could not employ research assistants and had to make do with what we had and do it ourselves.

Earlier research (not referenced, in order to maintain the anonymity of the research site) in the same Birth Centre and NHS trust had shown that a social model of birth that takes place within a local birth centre is one of the ways forward for midwifery. The appropriateness of the Birth Centre for realising the priorities for maternity care established in government policies was clearly expressed by the participating women and midwives, especially the need for a flexible, open-door service. The midwife participants in that study also expressed a need for mutual support from their peers, but especially from all managers within the trust. These same principles have been shown to be beneficial in other birth centre research studies (Kirkham, 2003; Walsh, 2007). We therefore sought to examine what had happened to make this same Birth Centre such a cause for concern.

AIMS OF THE RESEARCH

The research aimed to investigate midwives' and managers' experiences of the Birth Centre, which had opened in 2002 but was under threat of closure when the research started in 2006. Some of the difficulties and opposition experienced by the midwife who was seconded to help to set up this Birth Centre have been reported elsewhere (Shallow, 2003), and it is fair to say that the Birth Centre did not realise its potential. During the research process there was a real threat to its closure, with the facility only offering a 'nine to five' service. The 'open' or 'closed' status of the Birth Centre has changed frequently, and the unit finally closed in December 2007. This research therefore sought to examine the midwives' experiences of working within the Birth Centre, and the experiences of those who managed and those who were recruited to the facility, in order to better understand the chequered story of the centre.

This work attempts to provide an alternative perspective on birth centres to that given by the various and many narratives published on successful centres (Kirkham, 2003; Walsh, 2007).

ANONYMISATION OF THE RESEARCH SITE

In order to protect all those involved, we decided to anonymise the research site in order to protect the identity of the individuals involved. This was done in order to enable us to explore in detail a process that has occurred in many places. It is relatively easy to publish success stories, but stories of problems in maternity services are less commonly made public. We think that there is much that can be learned from such stories, but as they can be painful for all those involved, we wish to protect those individuals.

Interestingly, after presenting a conference paper on this research (Hughes *et al.*, 2008), we were approached by one local midwife who had correctly identified the site, and by five other midwives who thought that it could have been a place known to them (two of these were outside the UK). Clearly, then, the story that we tell in the following pages is not an isolated one.

One problem with anonymising the research site is that we cannot cite an earlier study which showed high levels of user satisfaction with the service provided there. We hope that we may be trusted in this regard, not least because a high level of client satisfaction is a usual finding with regard to birth centres (Kirkham, 2003).

NEGOTIATING ETHICAL HOOPS

Before we could start the research, we had to negotiate the various layers of ethical approval. We were aware that participation in research must be free and informed and that it should be made clear that there is no obligation to take part, and no penalty for declining to participate. Informed consent was obtained by means of a consent form, and withdrawal from the research was made possible at any point without incurring moral or professional judgement. One midwife who initially agreed to participate subsequently withdrew. As the data that were gathered would be put in the public arena, confidentiality could not be maintained because the words of the participants would be used to illustrate points made, and might be identified by others working locally. However, anonymity was a key feature of the research, with the site and all participants being anonymised, all names coded, and all tapes destroyed following data analysis. Data pertaining to specific places or people were dealt with sensitively. Previous research (Kirkham, 1999; Hughes *et al.*, 2002; Deery, 2005) has shown that participants often articulate past experiences that they have not disclosed previously. Relating some of these may be painful and distressing to the participants. Although it is not appropriate for the researchers to act as counsellors, the need for listening skills and acknowledgment of feelings was considered to be very important. The telephone contact numbers of suitable support services were also made available.

Approval of the study by the School Research Ethics Panel at the University of Huddersfield was relatively uneventful. Ruth Deery was invited to attend a meeting in order to answer various queries. Following the lengthy process of completing several forms for the NHS Local Research Ethics Committee, Ruth Deery and Deborah Hughes were invited to attend one of their meetings. We were asked, among other questions, how we would prevent bias, as we were clearly supportive of a birth centre approach! Notwithstanding the obvious differences in understanding and background with regard to research methodologies that this comment demonstrated, approval for the study was given.

METHODOLOGY

The study used the basic principles of a grounded theory approach, which is a specific systematic process of data collection, analysis and theory generation (Strauss and Corbin, 1998) that is non-linear. Data collection and analysis occurred simultaneously, and data were compared with all other items of data.

Data were collected via in-depth interviews with all of the midwives who worked at the Birth Centre and with important external individuals involved in the commissioning, steering and managing of the Birth Centre. An interview schedule was developed for each group of interviewees, which aimed to enable the participants to talk about their thoughts, feelings and conclusions about the Birth Centre in some depth. Themes from analysis of earlier interviews also informed subsequent interviews.

Financial constraints meant that these interviews were our only means of exploring what had happened in relation to this Birth Centre. The interviews were conducted as evolving discussions, with the three of us being able to probe the stories being told as appropriate to our developing analysis. In this way we were able to receive reflective, in-depth and prolific narratives, particularly from the midwives whom we interviewed, and we were both surprised and pleased that the data proved to be so rich in terms of providing insight into a struggling birth centre.

The interviews took place between August and December 2006. Key external players (health authority, local supervising authority and professional body personnel) were interviewed, together with five midwifery managers and 13 midwives. The interviews lasted between 25 and 120 minutes, and were all recorded with permission. Tape recorders malfunctioned during interviews with two of the midwives (Midwives 4 and 13), but extensive notes were made immediately after these interviews. The interviews took place at a time and venue of the interviewee's choosing. Three of the interviews (two 'externals' and one manager) were conducted by telephone, mainly due to problems of geographical distance, as these participants had either moved to different posts or retired and moved away. These telephone interviews tended to be shorter than those conducted face to face; all of the latter lasted at least 50 minutes.

All of the successfully recorded interviews were transcribed and the data were analysed using thematic analysis, identifying themes and cataloguing them through a three-stage process (Boyatzis, 1998). Stage 1 decided on design and sampling issues, stage 2 developed themes and a code, and stage 3 validated and used the code. Stage 2 consisted of three different ways to develop thematic codes, namely theory driven, prior data or prior research driven, and inductive or data driven (Boyatzis, 1998, p. 29). In this case the researchers used a data-driven approach, working with 'raw information' (Boyatzis, 1998, p. 30) from the transcripts. A process of regularly comparing data with those already obtained began, and as more findings (which became themes) began to emerge, a deeper analysis followed and the data were scrutinised for consistency and patterns.

In the next chapter the story of the Birth Centre unfolds.

REFERENCES

Boyatzis RE. *Transforming Qualitative Information: thematic analysis and code development.* Thousand Oaks, CA: Sage Publications, Inc.; 1998.

Deery R. An action research study exploring midwives' support needs and the effect of group clinical supervision. *Midwifery.* 2005; **21:** 161–76.

Hughes D, Deery R, Lovatt A. A critical ethnographic approach to facilitating cultural shift in midwifery. *Midwifery.* 2002; **18:** 43–52.

Hughes D, Deery R, Kirkham M. 'A poisoned chalice': midwives' experiences of a struggling *birth centre.* Paper presented at the International Confederation of Midwives (ICM) Triennial Congress 2008, 1–5 June 2008, Glasgow.

Kirkham M. The culture of midwifery in the NHS in England. *Journal of Advanced Nursing.* 1999; **30:** 732–9.

Kirkham M (ed.). *Birth Centres: a social model for maternity care.* Oxford: Books for Midwives; 2003.

Shallow H. The birth centre project. In: M Kirkham (ed.) *Birth Centres: a social model for maternity care.* Oxford: Books for Midwives; 2003. pp. 11–24.

Strauss A, Corbin J. *Basics of Qualitative Research: techniques and procedures for developing grounded theory,* 2nd edn. Thousand Oaks, CA: Sage Publications, Inc.; 1998.

Walsh D. *Improving Maternity Services: small is beautiful – lessons from a birth centre.* Oxford: Radcliffe Publishing Ltd; 2007.

CHAPTER 3

The story of the Birth Centre

THE EARLY DAYS

The Birth Centre that is the focus of this study, like many others set up in recent years, was born out of closure and reconfiguration of maternity services (Fraser *et al.*, 2003; Hall, 2003; Manero and Turner, 2003; Shallow, 2003). The town in which it is located originally had a separate maternity hospital, which opened after World War I, located across the town from the general hospital. This maternity hospital was closed in the early 1990s, and services were moved into pre-fabricated buildings, dating from World War II, at the general hospital. In 2001, that maternity unit was closed after lengthy public consultation, parliamentary debate and a long campaign to save it, and the town lost its full range of maternity services. The maternity unit in a neighbouring town now provided maternity care, although some women opted to give birth in another maternity unit 10 to 12 miles away.

During the period of public consultation preceding the closure, the health authority decided to explore the option of a birth centre, so that giving birth locally remained a choice for some women (Shallow, 2003). The acute trust, which was responsible for running the maternity services, was opposed to this plan. However, led by its consultant in public health, the health authority proceeded with a feasibility study and employed a midwife to work on this (Shallow, 2003). The feasibility study consulted widely and looked at a number of models. It strongly recommended a 24-hour birth centre staffed by midwives who were committed to a birth centre concept. The feasibility study was completed before the closure of the maternity unit, and was accepted by the health authority. Under some duress, and in the face of public support for a birth centre, the acute trust also accepted the plan, despite opposition from many trust managers, obstetricians and midwives. Operational meetings to progress the birth centre plan were initiated, and a midwifery manager was seconded to coordinate matters.

Midwifery opposition at grass-roots level appears to have been synonymous with opposition to the wider plan of closure and relocation of services. Although some midwives disagreed with the concept of a birth centre, most midwives were not opposed to the Birth Centre as such, but perceived support for it as backing down from their long-fought campaign to maintain a broad range of maternity services locally. They had campaigned for more than two years, been to Parliament, organised petitions and demonstrations, written letters and involved the media, and were not prepared to support a compromise, which was what they perceived the Birth Centre to be.

RECRUITING THE MIDWIVES

In late 2001, advertisements for Birth Centre midwives were placed in the local and national press, and in early 2002 a Birth Centre Coordinator was appointed on a G-grade (this grade was the equivalent of a 'Sister', i.e. a senior clinical midwife with responsibility for the care of a group of 'patients').

There had been considerable disquiet regionally among midwives about the low grading of this important post, and this issue will be discussed later. The first midwife to be appointed to this role resigned on her first day when it became apparent to her that the post would not be able to develop as she had envisaged (Shallow, 2003). The second coordinator, also a midwife with considerable experience and ability, was consequently appointed in February 2002.

During the spring of 2002, Birth Centre staff were appointed, but the centre did not open as scheduled, and these midwives (eight whole-time equivalents, who had moved to the area for these jobs and who were highly motivated) spent some months orientating to the mother unit and the community and doing various training courses. Healthcare assistants were appointed later. The Birth Centre finally opened in July 2002, but this was not marked by an official or formal ceremony; this issue will be returned to later.

The Birth Centre initially offered a 24-hour service staffed by two midwives and a healthcare assistant on most shifts, as envisaged in the feasibility study (Shallow, 2003). The staff had specifically chosen and been chosen to work in the Birth Centre, and were committed to the concept and to providing a woman-centred service in the town. The midwives took the initiative and began to provide antenatal care for many of the women who wanted to give birth at the Birth Centre. Postnatal care was offered at the Birth Centre, and the midwives went out to visit women in their homes in an attempt to extend continuity of care and promote their service, thereby fulfilling the plan for the Birth Centre which had been agreed and accepted by the stakeholders (Shallow, 2003). During the five months that the centre was open in 2002, a total of 54 women gave birth in the unit.

WIDENING CRACKS

By November 2002, only four months after the opening, the coordinator and three other midwives had left. The reasons for this will be discussed in more detail in the following chapters, but the central issue was a perceived and experienced inability to progress the development of the Birth Centre in the way that they had aspired to do. The midwives also appealed against their grading (F), as they were graded lower than their community midwifery colleagues (G). (An F grade was the equivalent of a staff grade with devolved responsibility for care of specific 'patients'. In the Clinical Grading Review of 1988, community-based midwives were expected to be at a minimum of G grade.)

A temporary coordinator was appointed, and the community midwifery manager took on overall management of the Birth Centre. The community midwives were relocated into the building at this point and ran the community midwifery service from there, although the two services were still being run separately at this stage. Also at this time (late 2002) there were many changes at senior management level in the trust. These changes occurred at a time when the Birth Centre was undergoing its own early crisis.

By March 2003, eight months after the Birth Centre had opened, no formal opening ceremony had been arranged. At the time of opening, the booking criteria had excluded women having their first baby, as it was felt by managers that the Birth Centre needed to run for six months with only multiparous women so that the midwives could settle into their 'new' practice. Again, by spring 2003 there was no progress with regard to extending the booking criteria to include first-time mothers. In May 2003, ten months after the centre had opened, three more of the original midwives resigned, including the temporary coordinator, and their posts were only partially covered by secondments of trust midwives into the Birth Centre. At the same time, healthcare assistants were removed from night shifts, leaving one midwife working alone at night, and the community midwifery manager took over the coordinator's remaining functions.

In July 2003, the Birth Centre celebrated its first birthday with a garden party, which was organised solely by the Birth Centre midwives. Although they were invited, none of the managers attended this event. The midwives had still not received the go-ahead to care for first-time mothers, and they now made another formal request for 'permission' to do so.

In late 2003, a new Chief Executive was appointed. The Birth Centre midwives' grading appeal was still ongoing, and their formal request to look after first-time mothers had still not been answered. They approached the new Chief Executive about the latter issue and were finally given permission in January 2004, 18 months after the opening of the Birth Centre. However, they had been visiting postnatal clients in the community up to this point, but were now stopped from doing so, as it was felt that there was duplication of travel between the Birth Centre and community midwives.

In the summer of 2004 there was a second birthday garden party, which the new Chief Executive attended, to the delight of the midwives. At the same time it was being mooted that the community and Birth Centre midwives would merge and the Birth Centre would be run as a 'closed unit' at night – that is, the Birth Centre would be unstaffed and locked at night. This meant that when a woman in labour telephoned the obstetric unit, the midwife on call would be rung and would meet the woman at the Birth Centre with the keys. This prompted the remaining Birth Centre staff to write a report arguing for the retention of a 24-hour service on financial as well as quality-of service grounds, making the point that on-call and call-out costs would be as high as the cost of staffing, and would provide a poorer service. Nonetheless, the Birth Centre was now being covered increasingly by community midwives working alongside the few remaining Birth Centre staff.

THE ROAD TO CLOSURE

In late 2004, despite the arguments against the move, the Birth Centre became a 'closed unit' at night, covered by a community midwifery on-call system, and the community and Birth Centre midwives were integrated, all now being (G-grade) community midwives.

By January 2005, 30 months after the opening of the centre, all of the original Birth Centre midwives who had been appointed from elsewhere had left. Postnatal stays were curtailed in order to reduce the cost of having an on-call midwife working. Women had to either return home a few hours after the birth to allow the midwife to go home, or be transferred to the obstetric unit 12 miles away.

In May 2005 the midwives organised an Open Day to try to publicise the Birth Centre to local women and families. However, by August 2005 the Birth Centre was closed from 5pm, and the evenings were also covered by on-call midwives. Any postnatal woman who was still in the Birth Centre when it closed at 5pm had to be transferred if she was not fit enough or did not wish to return home at that time. By the end of 2006, the Birth Centre had become a completely 'closed unit', opening only when a 'booked' woman was in labour, and remaining closed for many weekends when there were insufficient midwives to provide on-call cover.

This situation improved slightly in early 2007, when for a short period the Birth Centre was again open from 9am to 5pm. Two coordinators and a healthcare assistant were in post. They were organising drop-ins and 'look-and-book' tours in an attempt to increase booking numbers. However, this initiative was short-lived, and by April 2007 the centre was again a 'closed unit.' A healthcare assistant remained, whose role was to staff the unit from 7am to 4pm, to show women around the unit, to keep it stocked, and to call in a midwife if a woman was in labour. Other than this, the unit was covered for women in labour by the on-call community midwives. The number of births in 2007 was the lowest in the history of the centre (*see* Tables 3.1 and 3.2), and the Birth Centre closed at the end of 2007.

BIRTH CENTRE FIGURES

TABLE 3.1 Annual numbers of births at the Birth Centre

Year	Number of births
2002 (5 months)	54
2003	123
2004	207
2005	175
2006	190
2007	61

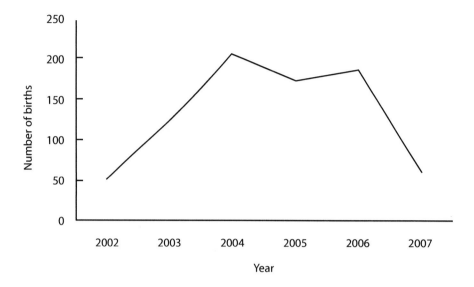

FIGURE 3.1 Births per year.

These data show the efforts made to increase bookings early in the history of the Birth Centre, and the falling off in the number of bookings when the organisation and staffing of the Birth Centre changed. This falling off occurred at the stage when a rise in the number of bookings would have been expected because sufficient women had already birthed there to influence local expectations about place of birth. We also know that these women were highly satisfied with the service.

TABLE 3.2 Annual numbers of transfers in labour from the Birth Centre

Year	Number of births	Number of transfers in labour
2002 (5 months)	54	Not available
2003	123	9
2004	207	42
2005	175	Not available
2006	190	64
2007	61	16

The figures for transfer in labour are interesting because they do not fit with the numbers of births. The figures for 2003 suggest that the Birth Centre midwives were confident in dealing with births in this setting. The considerable rise in the number of transfers relative to the number of births in 2006 and 2007 reflects the limited availability of the service, and the attitudes and morale of the staff concerned. The community midwives who were working there at that time were reported to be lacking in confidence in birth centre birth and to be 'so tired.' Many of them did not share the Birth Centre's philosophy (*see* Chapter 7). These changes in transfer rates were not linked to any changes in clinical outcomes, which remained good throughout.

No data are available for transfers in 2005. Our enquiries led to the statement that accurate figures for that year could not be found 'as there were four coordinators that year and the figures seem to have disappeared.'

TABLE 3.3 Annual numbers of neonatal transfers

Year	Number of births	Number of neonatal transfers
2002 (5 months)	54	Not available
2003	123	2
2004	207	1
2005	175	2
2006	190	2
2007	61	2

These figures are low, and no conclusions can be drawn from them.

TABLE 3.4 Annual numbers of postnatal transfers

Year	Number of births	Number of postnatal transfers
2002 (5 months)	54	Not available
2003	123	6
2004	207	10
2005	175	3
2006	190	8
2007	61	1

These figures are similarly low. The relatively high number of postnatal transfers in 2006 may reflect the limited opening hours of the Birth Centre at that time.

Tables 3.1 and 3.3 demonstrate the considerable midwifery effort from 2002 to 2006 that went into trying to make this Birth Centre a going concern. Recognition must be given to the midwives who worked hard to achieve the numbers that they did. Their story follows in the next chapters.

REFERENCES

Fraser D, Watts K, Munir F. Under the spotlight: Grantham's midwife-managed unit. In: M Kirkham (ed.) *Birth Centres: a social model for maternity care.* Oxford: Books for Midwives; 2003. pp. 39–52.

Hall J. Free-standing maternity units in England. In: M Kirkham (ed.) *Birth Centres: a social model for maternity care.* Oxford: Books for Midwives; 2003. pp. 3–10.

Manero E, Turner L. Users in the driving seat. In: M Kirkham (ed.) *Birth Centres: a social model for maternity care.* Oxford: Books for Midwives; 2003. pp. 63–70.

Shallow H. The birth centre project. In: M Kirkham (ed.) *Birth Centres: a social model for maternity care.* Oxford: Books for Midwives; 2003. pp. 11–24.

CHAPTER 4

The dream job:
niche practice in midwifery

Interviewing the midwives was interesting not only for what was said, but also for the way in which it was said. Pride, enthusiasm, pleasure and joy were revealed in the way many of the midwives reminisced or reflected on their experiences of the Birth Centre. This reinforced what was being said in words, and what those words spoke of was the importance of the Birth Centre to them as an opportunity to actualise their dream of midwifery:

> When I was offered the post . . . I was ecstatic, it was my dream job . . . true woman-centred care without any intervention or meddling. (Midwife 2)

> When I first got the job at the Birth Centre I felt as though all my Christmases had come at once . . . I felt it was my chance to practise as a true midwife . . . it was fantastic . . . it was right up my street. (Midwife 3)

The Birth Centre represented an ideal – the possibility of being able to be the midwife they had always wanted to be, and of practising as they had envisaged. This ideal practice appeared to have certain qualities, including autonomy, woman-centredness, a relationship focus, a shared philosophy, and quality care. It also valued the facilitation of natural birth and the midwifery skills that underpin it.

Walsh (2007) describes the birth centre in his study as a postmodern workplace, in which power is shared, bureaucracy is sidelined, and flexibility and adaptability predominate in an environment in which the woman and her individual physiology are at the centre. Walsh (2007) uses the term 'niche' in relation to the products of postmodern 'flexible' firms, and in relation to service industries such as health. We propose that it could equally be applied to service delivery in which the personal takes precedence over systems:

> They [the women] so appreciated every little thing that you did for them . . . I think it was a very high standard of care . . . it wasn't a conveyor-belt system. . . . It was family-orientated . . . it was responsive to the needs of the public. (Midwife 12)

> It was lovely . . . to be able to focus properly one to one on a lady. You revisit normal midwifery and you come across other aspects that you've never actually seen before, like water births, like a natural third stage . . . you get to believe that a woman can deliver a baby normally without interference. (Midwife 11)

AUTONOMY AND FREEDOM

Autonomy and freedom are central to the niche (Griew, 2003; Jones and Walker, 2003; Kirkham *et al.*, 2006). Walsh (2007) likens this to Freire's concept of 'praxis' (Freire, 1996, p. 47), whereby oppressed groups can realise their dreams through action. The midwives who were appointed to their 'dream job' expressed this dynamic towards self-realisation:

> They [the Birth Centre midwives] were all really, really supportive, really enthusiastic, really keen to promote woman-centred care. . . . To me, working in the Birth Centre gives you that freedom to practise being a midwife or more freedom to be a midwife. (Midwife 5)

> Clinically it was just lovely. I enjoyed every moment because I'm happy without doctors, and I'm happy making my own decisions, and I'm perfectly happy with women who are birthing physiologically, and clinically it was just my dream, it was my dream job. (Midwife 1)

SHARED PHILOSOPHIES

Commonality or a shared philosophy and approach are part of the ideal (Griew, 2003; Hunter, 2003; Kirkham, 2003; Kirkham *et al.*, 2006). Being able to express their personal values was integral to the 'dream job' for midwives (Walsh, 2007). This requires a degree of professional autonomy and flexibility which enables midwives to respond to women's needs, and which greatly increases midwives' job satisfaction (Kirkham *et al.*, 2006; Deery and Hunter, 2010). Midwives work closely together, and are dependent on each other for a large part of their working lives. Thus common values underpin a happy team:

> We all had the same aims and objectives and we wanted to make it a very woman-led service, a very home-from-home service on a very personal basis. (Midwife 3)

> Clinically we were like-minded . . . we were all of like minds so it was really easy to work with them. (Midwife 1)

Shallow (2003, p. 12) has described the importance of this commonality of values to the birth centre movement: 'The term "birth centre" is more than mere bricks and mortar – it represents a set of values and beliefs about birth.' This like-mindedness is both a prerequisite for and a result of working in an environment such as a birth centre. Kirkham (2003, p. 254) points out this circularity when she states that 'midwives who choose to work in new birth centres are also a special group, seeking to work within an accepting and positive culture.' In other words, they come together to create what they are looking for. This often appears to be more than many health trusts have bargained for, as it can lead to effective political resistance further down the line (Walsh, 2007).

This ideal of a shared goal led to good teamworking and keen commitment to the service:

> Everybody pulled their weight, everybody pulled together and that made the job more exciting, a lot easier. . . . A lot of us did extra shifts. We were very, very, very fluid in the way that we worked shifts to cover the unit, so that financially we could keep it going without having to spend too much money. (Midwife 3)

This loyalty and commitment is a feature of other birth centres (Waldenström, 2003; Walsh, 2007). Thus we can see that the niche job allows expression of personal, professional and collective values, and the blurring of the demarcation between work and personal lives. Walsh (2007, p. 68) has described how this fluidity and 'communitarian ethos' builds community and social capital, but how undervalued this is in bureaucratic and monolithic structures like the NHS, thereby placing ideal practice at odds with the monopoly employer in the UK.

THE DREAM JOB: NICHE PRACTICE

We suggest that the dream job, or the opportunity to practise in a niche set-up, is a widespread and important concept in midwifery and does not just involve birth centres. Other means whereby midwives may manage to realise their ideals can include specialist posts (teenage pregnancy, substance abuse, domestic violence, infant feeding), Sure Start posts (now largely ended), independent midwifery, posts in small experimental schemes (e.g. one-to-one midwifery posts), jobs in the various small midwife-led units dotted across the UK, and posts abroad. A large study by Kirkham *et al.* (2006) showed that niches which gave midwives job satisfaction varied, as do individuals, but a degree of professional autonomy and the opportunity to develop relationships with clients and colleagues were of key importance.

Some of the midwives who were interviewed moved on to other niche posts in Sure Start local programmes (SSLPs) or abroad. This demonstrates the importance of the philosophy and values underpinning these jobs to the midwives who aspire to them:

> I called in [at an SSLP] to have a look and the staff that were here were a lot like me but in a different profession. They felt that families and mothers were the centre of what was important, so I came here. (Midwife 1)

These 'niche posts' enable midwives to explore ways of giving woman-centred care. They represent social rather than medical models of care, and provide opportunities for autonomous and innovative practice and skill development. They facilitate midwives in channelling their keenness and commitment and developing their skills and expertise. They also involve a great deal of autonomy and independence, and the building of relationships with clients:

I'd always had an ideal that midwifery isn't carried out in hospital, but that was really the only type of midwifery that I'd been exposed to . . . so I decided to take it really just to widen my own skills and to develop. (Midwife 5)

I love it and I actually like delivering the women and, since I've been there, I've had so much experience, we've had water births which I hadn't any experience of before. (Midwife 9)

Although these types of posts are frequently under threat of loss of funding or other constraints, they are nevertheless niches in which many midwives shelter for periods of their careers. They may represent important ways of retaining midwives in the profession, especially those who do not subscribe to a medical model of care, or who value relationships with women highly (Walsh, 2007). Hallett has discussed the importance of his local birth centre (in Crowborough) in the retention of midwives locally (Hallett, 2003). There was evidence that the Birth Centre that we studied was playing a role in retaining midwives, too:

If they asked me to go and work on labour ward now, I would hate it, the way that it's set up at the moment, because it's just too medically orientated. I just don't feel I could go back to that kind of environment. (Midwife 7)

If you can find a place where you're allowed to practise how you want to practise. I don't know whether it'll have to be independent midwifery or another country . . . to be able to practise such birthing. (Midwife 12)

Managers seemed to recognise the importance of opportunities such as the Birth Centre in encouraging certain midwives to remain in midwifery, and to understand the motivation behind their seeking of such posts.

Midwives pick on a nice experience, there's enough going off to keep them interested but they're not the factory type . . . once you get to about five thousand deliveries it gets a bit factory-like . . . and then you come into retention issues. (Manager 3)

The importance of choice and a variety of opportunities and models of working for midwives, many of whom are mothers or carers, was summed up by one midwife, who warned of a monolithic approach to maternity care provision and employment:

> I think there needs to be a choice for women and a choice for midwives. It needs to be workable for midwives. I don't think it is useful to say that everyone is going to do team midwifery, because that won't suit most midwives . . . while their kids were little or while they were looking after their mum or whatever, so I think it needs to be flexible space. I think there needs to be lots of options so that midwives can find somewhere to work comfortably depending on what they can do, and women can choose what they want. (Midwife 1)

Moving from one model of midwifery to another can be challenging, and requires adaptation on the part of the midwife. Particularly difficult can be the transition from the busyness culture of larger maternity units (that is, the need to focus on throughput), or from a 'process mentality' (Walsh, 2007, p. 52), to focusing on the quality and individuality of care:

> Coming to the Birth Centre, I found it . . . quite slow and I found that a little bit frustrating . . . I was used to being busy all the time. One of the reasons for wanting to go to the Birth Centre . . . was to get better continuity, to see what childbirth is about when it's not medicalised. I found that it was really, really nice once I'd kind of wound down . . . I just found that really fulfilling to me as a midwife and . . . from the feedback we got from the women [they were] really enthusiastic about the experience that they were having. (Midwife 5)

Hunter (2003) argues that there is a close link between midwives having (or perhaps taking) time, and the giving of time to women to achieve normal birth. It seems that organisational behaviour and physiology have the potential to converge in birth centres to benefit the health and well-being of all involved. Hunter (2003, p. 241) calls this 'real midwifery', and it is closely linked to what we are describing as 'niche practice' here. Walsh (2007) describes the timescape in the birth centre that he studied as being different to that of mainstream maternity care. It has been advocated that lessons from the 'Slow Movement' (Honoré, 2004) should be absorbed into maternity service organisation to counteract its 'McDonaldisation' of maternity care (Garrett, 2008, p. 62).

Birth centres may therefore be as important for midwives as they are for women, enabling 'parallel processes of empowerment' (Porter and Tinsley, 2003, p. 37). They offer choice, continuity and control for midwives as well as mothers (Department of Health, 1993), and undoubtedly increase the retention of midwives in the NHS. As Kirkham (2003, p. 255) has stated, 'Birth centre practice is therefore important for midwifery because it demonstrates what is possible.'

Birth centres represent an aspiration which may help to retain not only those midwives who work in them, but also those who do not, by holding out to them hope in terms of future practice options. The evidence from these interviews suggests that such 'niches' increase the happiness of midwives, which, while important for retention, may also contribute to reduced sickness rates and overall long-term health, thus benefiting the NHS in other ways. Walsh (2007) found very low levels of sickness in his birth centre study.

> The Birth Centre is a wonderful place and I've been in it when it's been buzzing with women in labour and those midwives have been so happy. (External 2)

> It was lovely . . . I think that's something that you're never going to get ever again . . . it was a great place to work . . . it was such a lovely atmosphere. (Midwife 12)

The Birth Centre represented an ideal for the midwives who worked there. It was a niche in which they experienced a convergence of their deeply held values and beliefs and their practice, and achieved, albeit temporarily, a synthesis of ideas and actions, the personal and the professional:

> If my daughter got pregnant . . . I would want her to have a baby in that type of environment. (Midwife 11)

NICHE PRACTICE VERSUS THE ORGANISATION

The monolithic tendencies of the NHS mean that its institutions value systems, uniformity and conformity (Walsh, 2007). The demands of the Clinical Negligence Scheme for Trusts (CNST) are an example of this, as are the guidelines of the National Institute for Health and Clinical Excellence

(NICE). This widespread protocolisation of healthcare, which was discussed in Chapter 1, leads to tensions in areas such as maternity care where there is a simultaneous although contradictory drive towards individualised, client-centred care and efficient, standardised systems. As described above, niche jobs in midwifery are characterised by being client-centred, valuing relationships over systems, and being autonomous and innovative. This leads inevitably to a clash with the mainstream service at some level. Page (1997) has described this clash as a 'fear of excellence', where financial arguments are used to undermine midwifery initiatives that involve the kind of niche practice we are describing here.

· Walsh (2007, p. 39) has explored this issue in some depth, outlining the differences between traditional or Taylorist versus postmodern or post-Taylorist organisations and their relationship to technocratic and holistic models of birth (Walsh, 2007, pp. 91–4), and the problems encountered by many birth centres. We do not intend to repeat his insights, but rather to show how the story of this Birth Centre illustrates the tensions in maternity care that Walsh describes.

Although financial arguments always arise (and will be discussed later in relation to the Birth Centre), the tensions between the mainstream and the niche are often expressed in accusations of 'elitism' or a 'two-tiered' service (Beney, 2003; Fraser *et al.*, 2003; Kirkham, 2003; Walsh, 2007):

> There was a bit of a two-tier system: women who went to the Birth Centre had a fantastic centre . . . whereas other women don't have that level of care. (Manager 5)

> Most of them [midwives] would think if you're working in the Birth Centre, you're a bit of an elite. (Manager 4)

The 'elitism' is alleged by the mainstream with the implication that the niche is the top tier and the mainstream service is a second best. The odd thing about this is that the allegation of 'elitism' is a criticism rather than praise. In other words, the second best (as defined by the detractors of the niche) is valued because it is larger, familiar and has tradition on its side. By raising the issue of a two-tiered system, the critics of the niche (and we are not just talking about the Birth Centre here, but about any similar niche in midwifery) lay claim to protect the interests of the majority of women over those of the minority who receive the 'elite' service. Equity, which is a widely held value in healthcare, is used as an argument for the status quo, and against service improvements. Although supporters of birth centres see them as the gold standard for maternity care (Beney, 2003), others would prefer to see a more uniform 'silver' or even 'bronze' service:

> It would have been impossible to bring everybody's care up to that high standard, and it was a case of having some equity. (Manager 5)

> I think that there was a two-tier system . . . they [the women] preferred the Birth Centre, they could sit and chat with the midwives and have an antenatal that lasted, a really good service if you like, as long as they liked and they didn't have to wait. Whereas the majority were having 10-minute appointments and having to wait for ages. . . . That set up some friction between community and birth centre midwives because it was like an elite service that they were providing. (Manager 1)

Making structural adjustments in order to bring the niche back into the mainstream as much as possible (i.e. to bring it down a tier) is seen as good management practice:

> I feel it has to be integrated, that it can't be separate staff because when it was separate staff there was a two-tier system . . . I think that all women deserve the same level of care. (Manager 5)

This same manager had worked hard to dismantle the original Birth Centre staffing arrangements, presenting this as a common-sense approach. Although she recognised and even admired the different approach of the niche midwives, this had not prevented her from ensuring that they were integrated into the mainstream. Ultimately there was no room for the difference that the Birth Centre midwives represented in her view:

> Birth Centre midwives as well are often seen as a different breed of midwife by the majority of jobbing midwives, and I think that that's where the 'us and them' is bred from. The language is different that the two groups of midwives speak. One talks about supporting the women when they're giving birth, and one talks about delivering women and it's completely different. The philosophies are different . . . the cultures are different. (Manager 5)

This drive towards uniformity in maternity care provision is not unique to the British NHS. The Stockholm Birth Centre was subjected to a similar process whereby the mainstream took back control over staff and practice when it had the opportunity to do so (Waldenström, 2003). What the mainstream wants and will ensure that it gets are 'jobbing midwives.' Meanwhile, many of those midwives still yearn for that 'dream job.'

Another criticism of the niche is that it is uncooperative and non-conformist. Again these are qualities that are not valued in a monolithic culture, where there is only room for one service and one set of values:

> The Birth Centre midwives were trying to run a separate service from the community midwives. Well, you can't do that . . . you have to work together. (Manager 3)

Uniforms are often at the crux of this kind of conflict, representing as they do the corporate influence of the mainstream (Shallow, 2003). The issue of uniforms will be discussed more fully later (*see* Chapter 9), but clearly they are deeply symbolic of the centrifugal pull of the dominant culture:

> It was how the bosses were about uniforms . . . management weren't very happy about when we were actually out of uniform anyway. It was a struggle to get out of uniform . . . we didn't want that power imbalance . . . why would you have to wear a uniform when you were in a home-from-home environment? (Midwife 12)

Conflict is therefore an inevitable part of the niche as the struggle to resist the centrifugal force of the mainstream intensifies, and the dream begins to sour:

> So we had these really heated meetings [with management] which made for an unpleasantness, a general feeling of 'this is not how I want to work.' Going to work, looking after women in labour . . . all that was gorgeous, but it was very much marred by all the stuff that was going on around. (Midwife 1)

> It became such an oppressive place to work in a way . . . the atmosphere with the community [midwives]. I mean some of the community midwives were lovely, but then there were others, you just got the feeling . . . it became a very oppressive place to work. (Midwife 12)

Lack of support from the 'jobbing midwives' can be the final nail in the coffin for those in a niche, and for birth centre midwives this can be manifested as criticism about intrapartum transfers (Beney, 2003; Fraser *et al.*, 2003; Griew, 2003; Hunter, 2003; Walsh, 2007):

> I've been on the Labour Ward and there's been a transfer from the Birth Centre for whatever reason . . . 'blah de blah de blah, like what's the point in having it [the Birth Centre] if you're just gonna transfer somebody in?' (Midwife 12)

> I just think they [the obstetric unit] don't necessarily appreciate the fact that you are totally on your own with no support and none of the facilities that they have . . . they forget that we are also out here with these women, and if something is going wrong, or you're not sure if something's wrong, you can sometimes be made to feel a little bit 'Oh, can't you cope? Can't you manage?' (Midwife 9)

Another common criticism can be related to workload, and this may stem from the valuing in mainstream services of what Walsh (2007) has termed the 'busyness culture' that is prevalent in UK maternity services today. Fraser and colleagues (2003) have even reported managerial anxiety that midwives would become bored in the birth centre that they established in Grantham, presumably because the pervasive busyness of maternity care is so deeply entrenched that it is seen as almost essential to midwifery practice.

One Birth Centre midwife was painfully aware of the criticism levelled at herself and her colleagues with regard to workload:

> I don't think relationships between hospital midwives and Birth Centre midwives have blossomed . . . there was a lot of animosity with the Birth Centre midwives because 'they're sitting about doing nothing in lovely surroundings.' (Midwife 5)

There is a suggestion that this kind of intra-professional conflict may serve the purposes of the mainstream, or that the Birth Centre was sabotaged through passive neglect:

> There didn't seem to be any effort made to actually help the community midwives and the Birth Centre midwives to work together . . . seeing it from

> both sides . . . I can see why people have behaved as they do . . . I feel that somebody from a managerial [background] or with a wider vision should've been able to . . . do something to help people to work together rather than just letting it carry on and cause all this conflict. (Midwife 5)

There are certainly lessons for midwifery managers here, as well as for the profession and for health service policy makers. Midwifery has an ambivalent attitude towards woman-centred and 'low-tech' care, both aspiring to it and resenting it at the same time. Managers seem to have a similarly ambivalent attitude to their staff, both wanting them to fulfil their midwifery roles, work in new ways and meet women's expectations, and at the same time wanting them to get on with the unfulfilling job as it is for the majority of midwives (and women). And always in the background the tapping of the finance officers' calculators can be heard as they work out what sort of care can be afforded, irrespective of the evidence with regard to what is most effective or acceptable to women, or even what is government policy (Shribman, 2007). The latter point will be discussed more fully later.

REFERENCES

Beney J. A GP's perspective. In: M Kirkham (ed.) *Birth Centres: a social model for maternity care.* Oxford: Books for Midwives; 2003. pp. 95–104.

Deery R, Hunter B. Emotion work and relationships in midwifery: enhancing or challenging? In: M Kirkham (ed.) *The Midwife–Mother Relationship*, 2nd edn. Basingstoke: Palgrave Macmillan; 2010.

Department of Health. *Changing Childbirth, Part 1. Report of the Expert Maternity Group.* London: Department of Health; 1993.

Fraser D, Watts K, Munir F. Under the spotlight: Grantham's midwife-managed unit. In: M Kirkham (ed.) *Birth Centres: a social model for maternity care.* Oxford: Books for Midwives; 2003. pp. 39–52.

Freire P. *Pedagogy of the Oppressed.* London: Penguin Books; 1996.

Garrett EF. *The childbearing experiences of survivors of childhood sexual abuse.* PhD thesis. Sheffield: Sheffield Hallam University; 2008.

Griew K. Birth centre midwifery down under. In: M Kirkham (ed.) *Birth Centres: a social model for maternity care.* Oxford: Books for Midwives; 2003. pp. 209–22.

Hallet R. The Crowborough birthing centre story. In: M Kirkham (ed.) *Birth Centres: a social model for maternity Care.* Oxford: Books for Midwives; 2003. pp. 53–60.

Honoré C. *In Praise of Slow: how a worldwide movement is challenging the Cult of Speed.* London: Orion Books; 2004.

Hunter M. Autonomy, clinical freedom and responsibility. In: M Kirkham (ed.) *Birth Centres: a social model for maternity care.* Oxford: Books for Midwives; 2003. pp. 239–48.

Jones O, Walker J. From concept to reality: developing a working model of a stand-alone birth centre. In: M Kirkham (ed.) *Birth Centres: a social model for maternity care.* Oxford: Books for Midwives; 2003. pp. 79–88.

Kirkham M (ed.). *Birth Centres: a social model for maternity care.* Oxford: Books for Midwives; 2003.

Kirkham M, Morgan RK, Davies C. *Why Midwives Stay.* London: Department of Health; 2006. www.nhsemployers.org and www.rcm.org (accessed 5 December 2009).

Page L. Misplaced values: in fear of excellence. *British Journal of Midwifery.* 1997; **5**: 652–4.

Porter R, Tinsley V. The Wiltshire model. In: M Kirkham (ed.) *Birth Centres: a social model for maternity care.* Oxford: Books for Midwives; 2003. pp. 25–38.

Shallow H. The birth centre project. In: M Kirkham (ed.) *Birth Centres: a social model for maternity care.* Oxford: Books for Midwives; 2003. p. 12.

Shribman S. *Making it Better: for mother and baby.* London: Department of Health; 2007.

Waldenström U. The Stockholm birth centre. In M Kirkham (ed.) *Birth Centres: a social model for maternity care.* Oxford: Books for Midwives; 2003. pp. 143–59.

Walsh D. *Improving Maternity Services: small is beautiful – lessons from a birth centre.* London: Radcliffe Publishing Ltd; 2007.

CHAPTER 5

Opposition to the Birth Centre

ALLIANCE OF THE UNWILLING

The Birth Centre was not the brainchild of anyone involved in the maternity services, but of a public health consultant in the commissioning health authority. Although this was partly, indeed probably, mainly to secure agreement for the proposals for future service reconfiguration, the idea of a birth centre was also genuinely believed to have intrinsic merits by those senior health authority managers who spearheaded the proposal (Shallow, 2003). One of them recognised the problem of trying to establish a birth centre in the face of the merger and closure of a local full maternity service:

> That presents a challenge to those of us who believe that birth centres are a really good thing because you want to sell them 'on the nose' rather than on the basis of 'this is what you can have because we've taken something else away.' (External 4)

The idea won favour with many people in the local community, particularly politicians and women, who wanted to see women's option to give birth in the town retained once obstetric services moved elsewhere (Shallow, 2003). On the other hand, opposition to the idea was widespread in the local health service from the start:

> The [then] Chief Nurse objected strongly to a birth centre. . . . The Trust were very much against it and didn't want to support it at all. . . . The Consultants

didn't want the Birth Centre because they felt it was not the place for women to deliver. . . . The midwives that fought to keep the maternity unit open . . . didn't support the Birth Centre because it was a stand-alone unit. (Manager 1)

Opposition was clearly rooted in differing personal, political and professional perspectives, and was therefore complex in nature. However, this 'Alliance of the Unwilling' proved obdurate as well as pervasive, and underpins the subsequent history of the Birth Centre.

First, the Birth Centre was seen as being imposed from elsewhere, and the motives for this were questioned:

I'm not sure who 'they' are, but 'they' had to agree to promoting or facilitating some kind of birthing service in the area. (External 3)

The Birth Centre was an idea that I think came from government really as a way of appeasing the population . . . it had been forced upon the management, and even the management were going into it half-heartedly. It was brought about for the wrong reasons really. (Midwife 11)

An external midwife was employed on a secondment to undertake the feasibility study, and was employed by the health authority rather than the maternity service. This 'externalisation' of the project from the maternity services resulted in a range of problems that have been described elsewhere (Shallow, 2003), and meant that it proved difficult to get the Birth Centre established. It was compounded by the eventual need to employ mainly outside midwives to staff the centre, further disengaging local health professional investment in the Birth Centre.

Opposition to the Birth Centre was multi-faceted, and coalesced from many different perspectives, with serious consequences for the midwives working there and the service that the centre was attempting to offer women:

I felt like midwives that were on community didn't support the Birth Centre and neither did the GPs. . . . Women would come to the Birth Centre and say 'Oh my GP told me I couldn't come here, it wasn't safe' . . . the community midwives weren't telling the women about the Birth Centre because the women would say 'Oh my friend told me' or 'I've been to the midwife for weeks and she never mentioned this place'. So we knew there wasn't much support from the GPs, the midwives, or from the managers. . . . And then there were the consultants as well. (Midwife 1)

Where birth centres are seen as supplementing a full range of maternity care services, they can enjoy widespread support (Porter and Tinsley, 2003), but where they are seen as a tool for withdrawing services, opposition from professional groups in particular can develop into a serious impediment to success (Dolman, 2003). At Edgware Birth Centre, one of the best known and most successful birth centres in the UK, a strategy for dealing with resistance was built into its development (Dolman, 2003), but opposition was probably too pervasive with regard to the Birth Centre in this study for any such strategy to be developed or implemented effectively.

MIDWIFERY OPPOSITION

The reasons behind the considerable midwifery opposition to the Birth Centre are complex. The local midwives had fought a long campaign to save the full range of maternity services locally (Shallow, 2003). To them, the Birth Centre represented defeat and loss both for themselves and for local women:

> They [the local midwives] didn't want to change . . . they were very much tied up in . . . putting a fight on to maintain services as they were . . . they were very, very, very against the closure . . . because they felt that the women were getting a lesser service . . . the alternative of a birth centre wasn't a high priority. (External 2)

> I've tried to say to lots of them [midwives affected by previous closure] . . . 'I think you're bereft, I think you feel betrayed' . . . I think there's deep-seated unhappiness about the way they've been treated over the years . . . [they] just thought it was futile. (Midwife 1)

This profound sense of loss and bereavement does not appear to have been addressed at the time or subsequently, although the midwives' anger and behaviour are consistent with what we know of the processes of response to loss (Kubler-Ross, 1969). We found no evidence of any work ever having been done to acknowledge or mitigate these feelings. Instead they were left to transmute into sabotaging and gate-keeping behaviours with regard to the Birth Centre, with serious repercussions both for the centre and for the midwives working in it, as will be discussed more fully later.

These issues have implications for other services where birth centres are born out of closures and loss of services. Although we cannot offer any clear solutions, it does seem apparent to us that an investment of time and effort in acknowledging and addressing the 'losing' midwives' feelings and concerns is vitally important to the future of a service that is undergoing any kind of reconfiguration.

Most midwives who care about the NHS (and these are probably the majority of midwives) are likely to oppose, on both moral and professional grounds, any changes that they believe will disadvantage the choices and services available to local women. The midwifery ethos of service to women, which is so often relied upon by the NHS, demands this. The flip side of this is that those same midwives must be engaged with when those undesired changes take place. To expect quiet acquiescence is naive and fails to respect the very energy that maintains the service – the willingness of most midwives to make a personal and professional investment in a health service that is often understaffed and under-resourced. To our knowledge, no study has ever been undertaken in which the primary focus was the experience of staff in reconfigurations such as those which are currently widespread in maternity services. The undoubted impact of alienated staff on subsequent services warrants further investment in understanding staff responses and providing appropriate support.

Some of the local midwives in the area of our study were opposed to the idea of a birth centre, in keeping with a generally conservative position with regard to place of birth and ways of working:

> A lot of midwives felt that the Birth Centre didn't represent what they were fighting for. They wanted a proper maternity unit, not the Birth Centre, and a lot of midwives didn't agree with the Birth Centre as a concept. They didn't agree with home births, so they weren't going to agree with a birth centre. (Manager 1)

> It wasn't something that the midwives wanted. The midwives weren't playing ball. . . . It wasn't something that was welcome. (Manager 5)

> There wasn't the interest . . . from the hospital midwives to go and work in the Birth Centre because they hadn't worked in that model . . . it was quite a medicalised model they were used to. (External 2)

However, other local midwives were more interested in the idea of birth centres, but felt that professionally they were between a rock and a hard place, and unable to voice or act on their support for the concept, given their concomitant desire to maintain a consistent and collective position of opposition to the closure of the maternity unit:

> We'd fought tooth and nail, we'd gone on rallies, we'd gone down to London, we'd got petitions . . . so when the Birth Centre came about it was almost like if we went with the Birth Centre it was going along with the official stance of losing maternity services [in the town], and that's why there was resistance . . . it wasn't the idea of the Birth Centre, it was the end of a long battle . . . there were loads of [local] midwives who would have been ideal Birth Centre midwives who passed the opportunity up of going to the Birth Centre because it was a political argument initially. (Midwife 11)

Not only did the local midwives passively distance themselves from the Birth Centre, but also some of them acted as gatekeepers to the service, blocking women's potential choice of the Birth Centre for their care:

> The community midwives weren't offering it as an option to all suitable women. (Manager 5)

> There may have been some midwives around at that time that wouldn't offer it as an option. (Manager 4)

> The women that came, a lot of them were from word of mouth, a lot of them didn't seem to know it was there, it was one of those treasures that no one had heard about. (Midwife 8)

The lack of information given to women by those in a position to supply it effectively constrains choice for women, and is one of the ways in which healthcare professionals resist and control policies that are imposed on them (Kirkham and Stapleton, 2001). The Birth Centre midwives, who came from elsewhere and who had therefore not been part of the struggle to keep full maternity services in the town, were on the receiving end of this widespread gatekeeping, as were pregnant women:

> One of the things I felt quite frustrated about was the lack of people actually being referred to the Birth Centre . . . there was very, very little promotion around the Birth Centre . . . there was a lot of resistance from the local GPs as well and perhaps some of the community midwives . . . there just seemed to be a lot of politics around people keeping the women to themselves . . . they're not our women to keep, are they? (Midwife 5)

Withholding information, as described above, is one form of gatekeeping, but choosing what information to give and how to present that information is another effective way of constraining choice:

> Community midwives are the gatekeepers to birth centres . . . and I do know that we had midwives telling the women 'You can't have an epidural if you go in there' . . . and giving all the bad bits before the good bits. (External 1)

Although midwifery opposition was important in undermining the Birth Centre, as we shall see, many midwives did come to support it to some extent and, at the end of the day, they have been the group which until recently kept the Birth Centre open. This fact does tend to reinforce our earlier point that it might have been a sound strategy, much earlier in the process, to have invested more in addressing their initial ambivalence and getting them on board sooner.

GENERAL PRACTITIONER OPPOSITION

The extraordinarily resilient power base and independence of general practitioners (GPs) in terms of the wider NHS have a long history, and discussion of this is beyond the scope of the present work. However, it was clearly recognised as a problem with regard not just to this Birth Centre, but also to the birth centre movement in general (Beney, 2003; Fraser et al., 2003, Manero and Turner, 2003):

> We're moving over to practice-based commissioning consortia and the idea is that puts general practitioners much more again into the forefront in terms of commissioning decisions, which from the point of view of those of us who would like to see more midwifery-led birthing care . . . you don't relish the prospect really because general practitioners, on the whole, are pretty conservative in terms of their view about maternity care. (External 4)

General practitioner power, especially with regard to referral for care, is enshrined in health service protocols and bolstered by a mythologising of the past role of the GP, as indicated in the following quote:

> I remember meeting with some of the GPs who compared it with the old maternity homes and the horrendous things that went on then, you know like 30 years ago, and they still remember these things so they don't support the Birth Centre . . . we've even got a GP surgery that won't let the midwife refer women to the Birth Centre. All the women from that practice, they've got to be referred for consultant-led care . . . this is what you're up against all the time. (Manager 1)

We wonder exactly how many of these GPs really do remember maternity homes, and how extensive their experience of them was. Very few GPs who are still practising can have had much experience of maternity homes, most of which were already closed by the time the Peel Committee reported in 1970 (Tew, 1998). Furthermore, maternity homes were heavily influenced by the GPs in the locality who provided medical services to them, and who would have had daily access, and sat on their management committees. Indeed, GPs made submissions to the Peel Committee, albeit to no avail, in support of 'GP maternity homes' (Tew, 1998), presumably because they did not consider them quite so 'horrendous' at that time.

In terms of the gatekeeping of women described in the above quote, it appears to have gone largely unchallenged by the consultants who were, we must assume, accepting inappropriate referrals, and by the midwifery managers, who continued to supply recalcitrant GPs with midwives on those GPs' terms. It is therefore arguable that the power thus wielded by the GPs in this case is somewhat similar to the emperor's new clothes, dependent on collective collusion and illusion.

The midwives identified the financial underpinning of GP power as a factor in limiting choice for women and midwifery development:

> The other thing we were also up against was the GPs, and the GPs, whether we like it or not, have a lot of power because maternity services take money to them . . . if true midwife-led care came into that you can see they're going to lose money, and they don't want to do that. (Midwife 6)

In our experience elsewhere, the strategy most commonly adopted by midwives in the face of GP opposition is to try, usually with limited success, to persuade them of the merits of the midwifery position, and then to find ways of edging them out of the picture as much as possible. One of those involved felt that more should have been done at this level with regard to GP gatekeeping:

> There were a lot of meetings with GPs . . . to get them on side, to encourage them to refer the women to the Birth Centre but . . . those changes come slowly . . . so . . . you [should] bypass the GP, make the midwife first point of contact . . . those sort of initiatives need addressing to be able to do something about boosting the numbers. (External 2)

GPs in the town were insufficiently won over, but there appears to have been little or nothing done to bypass them, perhaps because of the midwifery ambiguity about the Birth Centre which was, as we shall see, compounded by managerial ambivalence and obstetric resistance. The following interviewee recognised the 'alliance of the unwilling' at work:

> We were able to persuade the Consultants far better than the GPs, and the GPs were so bad it just came to 'Well, we can't do anything about it', but I'm sure that if you had [community] midwives who had the same philosophy as the ones who were working in the Birth Centre, they would have worked on the GPs. (External 1)

Whatever their motives, GPs played an important negative role in the story of the Birth Centre, and that role was not effectively challenged either by the midwives or by those with greater financial and political control:

> Some GPs are a real barrier . . . there is nobody who can really tackle that you know, PCTs [primary care trusts] don't actually manage GPs. (Manager 3)

> Had they been able to be much more forceful, and I blame the health authority, with the group practice that were right next to the Birth Centre, who would have been so influential had they been positive, but sadly those GPs told women they would die if they went in there. So we had the greatest hostility from the practice that could have fed the largest group of women into that Birth Centre. (External 1)

To our personal knowledge, this kind of scenario is being played out elsewhere in relation to new birth centres. The perils of not addressing GP intransigence at the highest level are obvious – women are denied choice and birth centres are undermined.

OBSTETRIC CONSULTANT OPPOSITION

Birth centres are ideally an integrated part of a wider maternity service, and both support and are supported by the local obstetric unit and the colleagues working there to ensure optimal care and choice for women (Manero and Turner, 2003; Porter and Tinsley, 2003). The support of local obstetricians is essential for efficient and efficacious care when women are transferred between units, as will be inevitable. Good working relationships, based on open communication and trust, as well as mutually agreed protocols, underpin successful birth centres (Porter and Tinsley, 2003). Unfortunately, this was not the situation with regard to the Birth Centre in this study:

> If we ever wrote to the consultants for an opinion, they would write unpleasant letters back . . . and say 'Don't ask me for an opinion about whether this woman can give birth at the Birth Centre, I'm not giving you one.' (Midwife 1)

As with the midwives, obstetric opposition to the Birth Centre may have initially been congruent with the desire to retain a full range of services locally, although there seems to have been an element of opposition to the very concept of birth centres, regardless of what happened to the rest of maternity services:

> One particular consultant, who was very vocal at the outset about his opposition to the Birth Centre. . . . His influence in not wanting the Birth Centre was quite crucial. (External 3)

> This solution [the Birth Centre] was not, I have to say, initially welcomed with open arms by a number of people. The consultant obstetricians were always against the idea for a midwife-led birth centre, and fought quite strongly against it. (External 4)

At best, any small support that existed proved ambivalent and unlikely to nurture the trust and communication essential to success:

> The lead obstetrician said 'Oh yes, I'm all in favour of this, but the first time it goes wrong, don't look to me for support.' (Midwife 6)

One interviewee summed up the profoundly negative impact on the Birth Centre of the absence of collegial support:

> Without acute [trust] support for a birth centre, it cannot work in isolation because it's set up to fail . . . if you haven't got a good relationship with your obstetric and acute service then that can create fear, it can create barriers, and then ultimately can have an effect on safety . . . you've got to have a good relationship, and that wasn't there from day one. (External 3)

This is an important issue – birth centres can only be successful if they are regarded as partners by other parts of the maternity service, and if they can thereby rely on others and be relied upon in turn to provide optimal and effective care for their clients. The collaboration and support of the host unit, which is where most transferred women will be taken, is extremely important (Schmid, 2003). Establishing a birth centre in the face of intransigent and widespread professional opposition, as described above, is clearly jeopardising its potential. Another interviewee described how obstetric power continues to constrain midwifery services more widely, despite policymakers' support for midwife-led care:

> Ideally one would not define the need for a midwife-led birth centre against the provision of obstetric services. Ideally one would identify the need for midwifery services first and then identify the need for obstetric services second because, in my view, they quite clearly serve different groups. But the reality is that the need for midwife-led services will be defined against what's provided by obstetricians, and I think that's the reality of the world we're in. (External 4)

How this convergence of opposition to the Birth Centre was able to predominate becomes apparent when looking at management opposition to the Birth Centre.

MANAGERIAL OPPOSITION

The role of senior trust managers

As mentioned at the beginning of this chapter, the idea of the Birth Centre originated from outside the acute trust, and was at least partly in order to appease local people and politicians who were opposed to the closure of the maternity unit:

> The reasons for opening the Birth Centre were perhaps the wrong reasons . . . the Trust didn't support it and has never supported it, and it was therefore never going to get off the ground because no one really wanted it. (Manager 1)

Opposition went right to the top of the trust:

> There was the, not the last Chief Exec, the Chief Exec before who . . . didn't like the Birth Centre . . . and he wouldn't let it have an official opening and all these kind of things, and he made it known quite widely that he didn't support it . . . and at that time the Chief Nurse wasn't very supportive either. (Manager 3)

> The Clinical Director doesn't like it, he hates the Birth Centre. (Manager 3)

> It became apparent to me throughout the whole process that we were being blocked at every stage by the Acute Trust. (External 3)

This opposition meant that key decisions were made that were neither in the interests of the Birth Centre nor aimed to ensure its long-term success. The senior trust managers may have been forced by the health authority to accept the Birth Centre strategically, but they appear to have used their decision-making power to ensure that they would have tight control of it operationally. This is best illustrated by the fact that there was no delegation of operational power, and the low grading of Birth Centre posts reinforced dependency on the unsupportive hierarchy in the trust. The low grading (G) of the coordinator post, in particular, was seen by those involved at the time as deliberately disempowering and disabling:

> The trust was absolutely against it [the Birth Centre], and my first concern was appointing at such a low level, because they insisted that the manager post would be G, and F grades for the rest. (External 1)

> The main midwife was only on a G grade and the rest were F grades. I think that caused a lot of animosity . . . from that point of view, everybody thought 'Well, the grading is not right anyway.' So there was a lot of unrest about what they were being paid to work in the Birth Centre. (External 3)

> Also it [the coordinator's grade] wasn't an H . . . it was obvious it was an H-grade post . . . some of the things that they said as to why they couldn't pay for an H grade didn't stand up . . . things could have been so different. (Manager 2)

The impact of this grading was foreseen in that the coordinator was in a clinical rather than managerial grade, and too low in the hierarchy to influence key policy and strategic decisions:

> A G-grade midwife running the Birth Centre would not get to any of the key meetings to have a voice and an influence as to how the Birth Centre would run. (External 3)

The inevitable result of this situation was that the coordinator left four months after the Birth Centre opened. Thereafter the Birth Centre midwives were managed by the trust midwifery managers, thus resulting in extra work for managers whose attitude to the Birth Centre was at best ambivalent.

THE ROLE OF MIDWIFERY MANAGERS

Midwifery managers, positioned hierarchically and philosophically between the trust and the midwives, were only too aware that they were in a difficult or even impossible position. The then Head of Midwifery was remembered by a number of interviewees as having recognised this:

> When she [the then Head of Midwifery] was given the job to oversee the Birth Centre, she walked on to the Labour Ward and one of the Birth Centre midwives who worked there heard her say it – 'I've been handed a poisoned chalice.' (Midwife 2)

I heard what the comment had been when she'd been given the project to lead, I was very sad to hear that – 'I've drawn the short straw' – that's the Head of Midwifery being given a project for midwifery-led care. (Midwife 6)

Clearly the situation was also a difficult one for midwifery managers further down the hierarchy who inherited the 'poisoned chalice':

I feel we're always playing catch-up really because we're paying for the mistakes of the past to a certain extent, and also lack of trust support for it. (Manager 3)

This ambivalence of the midwifery managers was recognised by the Birth Centre midwives, who appear to have found it harder to deal with than the outright opposition of those higher up in the trust hierarchy:

For the managers, the Birth Centre was there and they had to tolerate it . . . it was there and they had to just put up with it really, and I feel that had they been more pro-Birth Centre, rather than just tolerating it, I feel it would've been completely different. (Midwife 5)

That the midwifery managers ultimately toed the trust line is shown by the fact that they maintained a personal distance from the Birth Centre when they had a choice:

There was a garden party to promote the Birth Centre . . . and not one member of management turned up or . . . didn't appear to have sent any 'good luck' or 'hope you do well.' There didn't seem to be any kind of support whatsoever . . . that hurt an awful lot when none of the management bothered to turn up and show any support. (Midwife 5)

We had a big garden party . . . but not one [manager] came . . . and that was a massive blow for all the staff because all we wanted was a bit of recognition. (Midwife 3)

The importance of managerial support at all levels for staff who are working in an exposed situation outside of the mainstream is clearly important, as is shown by the same midwife's reaction to an albeit brief visit by the trust Chief Executive at a subsequent event:

> The following year we had again a lovely garden party, it was really fabulous and . . . the Chief Exec came which was lovely . . . he just came for half an hour and he said hello to everybody and off he went. But that to us was quite good. (Midwife 3)

The 'corporatisation' of professional managers that was evident here is often difficult for front-line staff to accept, as it represents a schism in previously shared professional values and commonality of outlook and priorities. These managers may continue to have the words 'midwife' or 'midwifery' in their job titles, but they are expected to dampen down or constrain the aspirations and demands of their fellow midwives arising from the core values of midwifery, so that they comply with corporate strategy and financial budgets:

> It was difficult to be in the position of being a manager of a service and being a midwife as well . . . you have a budget to balance and you want to have this other service going. (Manager 4)

The ambivalence of midwifery managers about the Birth Centre meant that they maintained a certain distance from the staff. They did not attend any of the various open days or fetes, as already mentioned, but their ambivalence also meant that they were unable to give any effective support to staff on a more day-to-day basis:

> A bit of recognition for the hard work wouldn't have gone amiss, but nobody once turned round and said to any of us 'You have done a good job' . . . we were battered all the time. (Midwife 2)

> I don't feel that I got the help and the support I needed to be able to do my job. (Midwife 3)

The lack of a midwifery managerial commitment to the Birth Centre meant that the service was kept in a kind of limbo, neither being driven forward by those in a position to help it, nor being openly opposed due to the political sensitivity of the issue. One interviewee summarised how the midwifery managers' attitude was interpreted by staff:

> I think it was just seen as a thorn in their side, and 'Really we don't want it, if it's got to be there then we'll tolerate it, but that's as far as it's going to happen.' (Midwife 5)

One external person involved described this as akin to paralysis:

> They [the acute trust] did not support the notion of a birth centre and were actually very opposed to it. . . . She [the Head of Midwifery] was paralysed because although personally she supported it, publicly she could not do so, so that was very, very difficult. (External 3)

This speaks volumes about the managerial culture in the NHS. It raises questions both about professional autonomy within that culture, and about NHS accountability to commissioners and the local population. As one interviewee pointed out:

> Although in principle commissioners can decide what they want and then commission it, in practice it's a mixture of commissioner intent and provider willingness to provide. (External 4)

Front-line staff are often accused of sabotage by managers, but it is clear that such behaviour can pervade an organisation such as an NHS trust.

PROFESSIONAL DISSONANCE IN MIDWIFERY MANAGEMENT

The midwifery managers' inability to integrate their personal and professional values and beliefs into their managerial role was pervasive. Reflecting on their words and actions, as discussed above, it seems to us that the trust's midwifery managers were experiencing what might be called *professional dissonance*.

By professional dissonance, we mean trying to hold simultaneously two, often conflicting, sets of values, namely the professional values of midwifery in which the managers have been educated and practised, and the values of the target- and star-rating-driven 'new NHS.'

Midwifery values include such notions as woman-centredness, individualised care, attention to psychosocial needs, one-to-one care in labour, continuity of care, and normality of childbirth. All of these presuppose a flexible, well-resourced and personalised approach to care. The managerial values of the new NHS, on the other hand, demand a systems-based approach of discrete targets, which emphasises certain measurable elements of care (e.g. antenatal screening uptake), clinical governance with its industrialised approach to risk management, and demand for ever more paperwork (the primary aim of which is to facilitate audit trails) and tight financial controls. The focus of managerial 'care' is the smooth running of the industrialised system to meet the requirements of the Clinical Negligence Scheme for Trusts, the Department of Health's various star ratings and, more recently, Care Quality Commission (CQC) scrutiny. Therefore the focus on the individual woman, which is so central in midwifery philosophy, becomes secondary to the outcome-driven values of NHS bureaucracy. Midwifery managers straddle this unhappy divide, and the duality of values that this creates is often experienced by clinical midwives as ineffectiveness or hypocrisy:

> I just felt betrayed. (Midwife 1)

> I don't want to work for people like that who just want to lie to me. (Midwife 2)

A birth centre represents a destabilisation of the path trodden by midwifery managers, as it challenges the supremacy of the medico-techno-bureaucratic values outlined above (Walsh, 2007), in which midwifery managers are immersed for most of their working weeks. It threatens to undermine the two main tenets of the new NHS, namely that care must be tightly controlled and as cheap as possible. As described in Chapter 4, a birth centre represents a midwifery ideal – family-centred, natural birth. However, the everyday management of a birth centre could reinforce the dissonance experienced by midwifery managers in that a birth centre demands the supremacy of midwifery values, and very few managers are currently able to deliver on this (Walsh, 2007). Even those who are able to do so experience considerable difficulty. Page (1997) describes a tendency of midwifery managers to opt for 'halfway models.' These, she states, are created to pay lip service to government policy and create an illusion of change, when in fact there is a 'constant resistance to success' (Page, 1997, p. 652). Such halfway models may nonetheless do much to relieve the personal unease caused by managers' 'professional dissonance', even if they ultimately do little for women or clinical midwives.

Success as a manager in the new NHS may therefore be largely dependent on not having midwifery values that are so strong as to interfere with the ability to toe the corporate line. This often creates a schism between the roles of management and leadership, as the latter is dependent on the expression in action of personal values. Walsh (2007) regards the ability to combine both roles as rare, but important to the success of initiatives such as birth centres. With regard to birth centres, Walsh suggests that few midwifery managers are able to provide leadership because 'the vast majority . . . have been promoted from within the acute maternity services model' (Walsh, 2007, p. 36). This issue was recognised as important by one of the managers whom we interviewed:

> You need that passion and that drive in the leadership. (Manager 5)

Appointing grade-F and grade-G midwives to work in the Birth Centre was, for managers experiencing professional dissonance, almost the sensible course of action because this sent out a message that leadership would be provided, if only on a clinical level, and at the same time would not interfere with managerial functioning. It can be seen as an unconscious admission that leadership could not be provided simultaneously with management, as values diverge. Inevitably, however, leadership without managerial power can achieve little.

The tension between two sets of professional values is what we name professional dissonance. Midwifery managers' resulting feelings of powerlessness have been described in a previous national study (Curtis *et al.*, 2003). We suggest that this has a personal cost for midwifery managers, and that they develop coping mechanisms when they experience powerlessness and loss of agency resulting from any persisting midwifery values that they hold. There are midwifery managers who embrace midwifery values and work with the explicit aims of fostering a social model of care and continuity of midwifery care, which birth centres are well placed to provide (Brodie and Leap, 2008). Such managers seek to transform midwifery services (Page, 2008). The managers in this study provided no evidence of such values. They had not sought to create a birth centre, but rather they had had a birth centre thrust upon them.

There was no clear support for the Birth Centre from anyone in a position to support it effectively, apart from one of the several chief executives who were in post during its short history. It has had no obvious champion since the health authority personnel who had instigated it moved on shortly after its opening. Conversely, there was widespread opposition by a range of powerful professional and managerial interests, the combined resistance of whom was not going to be overcome by a small group of low-graded midwives. This opposition could be seen as an 'alliance of the unwilling', uniting groups (GPs, obstetricians, midwives and trust managers) who more often have differing perspectives on the priorities for service improvement. The effect of all this was that the Birth Centre was undermined from the start:

> It's never functioned as it was intended to function . . . probably looking back, was it idealistic? But I don't think so . . . but it's not running as it was intended to run and it comes down to the fact that they never had strong support to begin with. (Manager 2)

The impact of this on the midwives working in the Birth Centre will be explored in the next chapter.

REFERENCES

Beney J. A GP's perspective. In: M Kirkham (ed.) *Birth Centres: a social model for maternity care*. Oxford: Books for Midwives; 2003. pp. 95–104.

Brodie P, Leap N. From ideal to real: the interface between birth territory and the maternity services organisation. In: K Fahy, M Fourier and C Hastie (eds) *Birth Territory and Midwifery Guardianship*. Sydney: Books for Midwives; 2008. pp. 149–69.

Curtis P, Ball L, Kirkham M. *Why do Midwives Leave? Talking to managers*. London: Royal College of Midwives Publications; 2003.

Dolman S. Trusts in partnership – professional collaboration. In: M Kirkham (ed.) *Birth Centres: a social model for maternity care*. Oxford: Books for Midwives; 2003. pp. 89–94.

Fraser D, Watts K, Munir F. Under the spotlight: Grantham's midwife-managed unit. In: M Kirkham (ed.) *Birth Centres: a social model for maternity care*. Oxford: Books for Midwives; 2003. pp. 39–52.

Kirkham M, Stapleton H (eds) *Informed Choice in Maternity Care: an evaluation of evidence-based leaflets*. York: NHS Centre for Reviews and Dissemination; 2001.

Kubler-Ross E. *On Death and Dying*. New York: Scribner; 1969.

Manero E, Turner L. Users in the driving seat. In: M Kirkham (ed.) *Birth Centres: a social model for maternity care*. Oxford: Books for Midwives; 2003. pp. 63–70.

Page L. Misplaced values: in fear of excellence. *British Journal of Midwifery*. 1997; 5: 652–4.

Page L. Being a midwife to midwifery: transforming midwifery services. In K Fahy, M Fourier and C Hastie (eds) *Birth Territory and Midwifery Guardianship.* Sydney: Books for Midwives; 2008. pp. 115–29.

Porter R, Tinsley V. The Wiltshire model. In: M Kirkham (ed.) *Birth Centres: a social model for maternity care.* Oxford: Books for Midwives; 2003. pp. 25–38.

Schmid V. Birth centres in Italy. In: M Kirkham (ed.) *Birth Centres: a social model for maternity care.* Oxford: Books for Midwives; 2003. pp. 161–72.

Shallow H. The birth centre project. In: M Kirkham (ed.) *Birth Centres: a social model for maternity care.* Oxford: Books for Midwives; 2003. pp. 11–24.

Tew M. *Safer Childbirth: a critical history of maternity care,* 2nd edn. London: Free Association Books; 1998.

Walsh D. *Improving Maternity Services: small is beautiful – lessons from a birth centre.* Oxford: Radcliffe Publishing Ltd; 2007.

CHAPTER 6

The experience of the Birth Centre midwives

WORKING IN A FRAGILE SERVICE

The experience of the Birth Centre midwives was of working in a fractured service with little support either for the Birth Centre itself or for the midwives staffing it. This had an ultimately devastating effect both on the service itself and on many individual midwives, leading the majority of them to leave within the first two years:

> The issue is it's a very fragile service. (Manager 3)

Their experience of the Birth Centre was to leave some of the midwives in a fragile state themselves. Walsh (2007) describes how working in an unsupported birth centre can be experienced as organisational bullying, and many of the midwives who were interviewed in this study seem to have experienced it as such. One midwife wept throughout her interview as she recalled her time at the Birth Centre, and many were visibly upset at times as they described the experience. One interviewee summed up the impact of working at the Birth Centre on the midwives:

> A lot of sadness. An awful lot of sadness and quiet despair. (External 2)

How the Birth Centre came to have this effect will be explored in this chapter.

RECRUITING FROM 'OUTSIDE'

Nearly all of the midwives were appointed from outside the area, so had little idea of the background to the Birth Centre and what they were getting themselves into when they accepted the jobs:

> We needed midwives who were committed to the Centre's principles because we hadn't that commitment from the [local] midwives because they were still grieving the loss of their maternity unit. . . . They got outside midwives . . . and they were all committed, experienced midwives who totally wanted to make the Birth Centre work. (External 3)

These appointments were very much driven by the Health Authority Working Group that was set up to drive forward the Birth Centre. The trust and midwifery managers therefore inherited a number of newly appointed and idealistic midwives who had no idea of the opposition or, at best, ambivalence of their new employers and managers with regard to the Birth Centre. The awakening of the midwives to their situation was therefore bound to be a painful one. Some of the midwives later described how they felt themselves to be pawns in a game:

> I started going to meetings about the Birth Centre and became increasingly cross about the whole thing because I just felt like we were misrepresented and people weren't listening to the Birth Centre and how it worked. (Midwife 1)

The midwife who was initially appointed to the post of Birth Centre coordinator resigned on her first day, partly in response to the grading of the post and partly because of how she foresaw things developing as a result of that low grading (Shallow, 2003). Unlike the other Birth Centre midwives, she had been involved in the setting up of the Birth Centre, and so was more aware of its context and history. Her moment of epiphany came during a uniform fitting:

> It was clear to me that the coordinator would have very little influence over how the facility would be run. . . . I felt I would be starting the job not with one hand tied behind my back, but with both, firmly secured. (Shallow, 2003, p. 23)

The other midwives, finding themselves in a difficult situation, tried initially to make the most of the opportunities that they believed the Birth Centre offered them and their clients:

> I kind of knew there was unease but when I first arrived, when I got the job, I didn't really ask how long the contract was or how long the Birth Centre was going to be open because, to be honest, I was so glad to go to a birth centre, I didn't mind if it only lasted a year. (Midwife 1)

This approach had some success, and there were many positive experiences, especially early on. However, from the beginning it was clear that the midwives were going to struggle to make the Birth Centre a success, and even early enthusiasm and experiences were shadowed by struggle:

> It all sounds very negative; it wasn't. I did have some good experiences and I worked with some fantastic, innovative midwives who did their best to promote the Birth Centre, to get it to work, to put a positive face towards the GPs. (Midwife 6)

ISOLATION AND FRUSTRATION: PAIN AND POWERLESSNESS AT WORK

Recognising that there was little support at a high level for the Birth Centre, one strategy that the midwives tried was just getting on with the job without reference to the wider maternity service:

> What marred it really was that we spent the whole time fighting really to be left alone, for them to leave us working how we were working, so I think that spoiled it really. (Midwife 1)

> We were not part of the decision-making process at all. We were kept firmly out of the loop because God forbid that we knew too much. (Midwife 2)

The pervasive lack of communication caused a sense of isolation and almost a siege mentality among the Birth Centre midwives:

> We were just sort of kept a lid on and a lot of that seemed to be lack of information . . . we all felt there was a bit of a hidden agenda . . . [gives example]. . . I knew nothing about it at all and I was furious . . . why didn't somebody just let us know? . . . it was the old mushroom thing, you know, keep them in the dark. (Midwife 3)

> Things all seemed to come through the back door rather than the front door; we always heard about them last. (Midwife 12)

The midwives became increasingly frustrated, feeling that they were being forced into confrontational situations that were not of their making:

> I went to quite a few meetings to try and stop it [the cessation of 24-hour staffing], but it was 'fait accompli' . . . by the time they were actually consulting with us I think it had already been finalised, and you were banging your head on a brick wall basically. There was no point. You just made a name for yourself as being somebody who stood up for the rights of women really. (Midwife 12)

This metaphor of banging one's head against a brick wall was repeated in the same or similar language by other interviewees. It is a very telling metaphor, as it conveys frustration, pain, futility, powerlessness, conflict, and a sense of not being listened to:

> I think motivation was going . . . I just felt as though I'd got a massive lump on my forehead from banging my head against a wall the whole time. (Midwife 3)

Another midwife also described the frustration of working at the Birth Centre, using similar language:

> All the time there seemed to be stumbling blocks . . . I did some waterbirth guidelines . . . they ended up going through after about 18 months, and everything took just such a long time to get anywhere, even one step forward . . . we got it all the time, constantly; I suppose the words that I want to say are 'beat us down.' (Midwife 3)

The following midwife makes the connection between blocking behaviours and power explicit:

> Every time we wanted to do something, we had to jump through so many flipping hoops . . . we were the Birth Centre midwives, we knew what needed to be done, yet no one ever listened to us . . . it was awful . . . she [the Birth Centre coordinator] felt she had no support. She had support from us lot but not from where the power was. (Midwife 2)

The midwives felt that they had no real involvement in the decision-making process in relation to the Birth Centre, or any understanding of that process. The feeling of being subject to conspiracy by others understandably took hold:

> I remember being at various meetings and suddenly finding out things. I think, well hold on a minute, I'm supposed to be the coordinator of this Birth Centre and decisions are being made and taken in rooms where I'm not present, and I'm finding out around a table, and it makes you feel stupid. (Midwife 6)

One of the areas in which the midwives encountered difficulties was being allowed to accept first-time mothers for Birth Centre care, an issue that has been reported for other birth centres (Fraser *et al.*, 2003). Initially the midwives had been told that they should not accept women having their first babies for the first 6 months after the Birth Centre opened, but when the time came to review this policy, no decision was forthcoming from managers. This state of affairs continued for a further year, until a new Chief Executive came into post and one of the Birth Centre midwives had the opportunity to bring this matter to his attention:

> Next EDG [Executive Directors' Group] he said why can't the Birth Centre take primips? Everybody looked at each other and said 'We don't know', and he said, 'Right then, they can do it.' And that was it, simple, five minutes but it had taken the rest of them a year . . . it's pathetic. They couldn't organise a piss-up in a brewery . . . so you know really it was the whole bag of lies and deceit and . . . nobody being honest with us. (Midwife 2)

It is noteworthy that this simple clinical operational decision was only finally resolved by the most senior non-clinical manager in the trust. This conversation between an F-grade midwife and the Chief Executive resolved an issue that none of the intermediate levels of management was willing to decide.

The frustration felt by the midwives about the organisational aspects of their working lives contrasted with the quality and enjoyment of their clinical experience. This made for a somewhat ambivalent work experience, as summarised by one midwife:

> We were so pleased because . . . we'd beaten the targets, we'd got an excellent safety record, we'd had women coming from here, there and everywhere wanting to have their babies with us, and the feedback, the satisfaction from these women . . . was wonderful. But it was as though we were kept down . . . we were kept in our place . . . we couldn't develop in the way we felt we ought to be able to develop, and there were a lot of very negative attitudes towards the Birth Centre and also, in some ways, towards the midwives who were there. (Midwife 3)

However, the organisational constraints under which the midwives were working did affect their clinical experience, as they found themselves unable to influence policy making and exercise their clinical judgement fully:

> We were trying to give midwife-led care and that was always frustrating because we were only allowed to give care that the obstetricians felt that a midwife could give . . . my training enabled me to look after pregnant women and to be able to make a clinical decision, and to refer on appropriately . . . we were never given that autonomy. (Midwife 6)

This midwife identified a lack of trust as key to the attitudes that she encountered. She felt that there was no trust in the midwives' clinical abilities or judgement, and that therefore they were not given the autonomy necessary for the job that they had been asked to do:

> You know, these midwives have all undergone training, they were all enthusiastic. Not one midwife in the unit would want to put a woman, a baby, a family at risk . . . you've got to be enthusiastic because, you know, sadly, in this culture at the moment, that the odds are against you . . . and I just wish there would have been total support, total trust in midwives. . . . Midwives were not allowed to manage the unit, midwives were not allowed to judge. (Midwife 6)

Although it quickly became apparent that there was a pervasive lack of support for the Birth Centre, the midwives tried to make the Birth Centre a success despite this:

> We'd done everything. We'd had banners printed which got stolen, we'd had promotion in the press, we did everything. We had a garden party every year, open days; we did everything because we wanted the women to come through the doors. (Midwife 2)

Walsh (2007, p. 31) also describes how a sense of being subjected to 'a tactic of "grinding down"' was reported by the midwives in the birth centre that he studied. Walsh's participants, despite working in a successful birth centre, experienced this grinding down as being manipulated by middle managers who were themselves being used by faceless power brokers further up the hierarchy, a situation that has clear parallels with that described here. Walsh (2007) also discusses how being under threat can become a way of life for birth centre midwives, and that the experience of this is deeply personal, as we have also found.

However, for the midwives whom we interviewed, optimism turned to despair and anger as they realised their inability to influence the situation, and that they were fighting a battle they could not win:

> There were a few of us that were keen to do everything to keep the Birth Centre the way it was and to keep it open . . . everybody felt from the very beginning that they were trying to close it, but I was always kind of optimistic . . . and everybody kept saying to me 'They'll let you down, don't believe them, they'll let you down.' . . . So I was ever optimistic, but sadly let down by them [management]. (Midwife 1)

This sense of being let down was felt on a personal level, and has been enduring. The midwives had been recruited on the basis of their energy, enthusiasm and vision, but once they were in post those qualities became problematic both for the midwives and for their managers. Most of the interviewees expressed an ongoing feeling of anger about what had happened, and had experienced a loss of trust in managers that they still felt at the time of the interviews:

> I just felt betrayed. I just felt we'd been misled, unsupported and a million other different negative adjectives I could think of; they're just not pleasant. (Midwife 1)

> My biggest disappointment was the management. (Midwife 6)

> What I don't like is people lying to me because it infers that I am an idiot and I don't know what is going on, and I don't want to work for people like that who just want to lie to me. (Midwife 2)

It was clear from the interviews that many of the midwives continued to be deeply affected several years later by what had happened to them at the Birth Centre. It is possible to surmise that their negative experience will continue to affect their attitude to health service management in particular for some time. Most of the midwives had left not only the Birth Centre but also the NHS trust as the situation worsened (seven midwives resigned within the first 10 months), and other trusts will have inherited the midwives' understandable cynicism and demoralisation, and other midwives will have heard them talk about their experiences. It is beyond the scope of this study to explore how this loss of trust and sense of betrayal affects the wider maternity service in the longer term, but this issue is of concern, given that midwifery is dogged by problems of retention and morale (Ball *et al.*, 2002; Kirkham and Morgan, 2006; Kirkham *et al.*, 2006).

BATTLE BY ATTRITION: THE OPERATIONALISATION OF NON-SUPPORT

Opposition to the Birth Centre has been described at length in the previous chapter. Alongside active opposition, there is also its passive flip side, namely non-support:

> She [the Birth Centre coordinator] didn't seem to have support from anywhere else. There didn't seem to be any proper line of management . . . there didn't seem to be any infrastructure to support the Birth Centre. (Midwife 5)

It can be harder to identify non-support than outright opposition, as non-support works by default through inaction, passivity and silence. Some of this non-support can be seen in the lack of communication and absence of facilitative management outlined above. The vacuum left by lack of support is quickly filled by a culture of inert chicanery:

> It was very, very clear to me that they were all playing some kind of political game . . . the Chief Executive . . . you could see in his eyes 'Where is this coming from? I didn't know this', I was being led astray . . . but we battled on. (External 3)

The lack of a formal opening was seen by many of those who were interviewed as indicative of the pervasive non-support for the Birth Centre:

> They needed help . . . from the trust to promote it and that wasn't forthcoming . . . they let those midwives down because it should've had its formal opening, it should have been celebrated and there should've been a lot more publicity. There should've been the website, there should've been all sorts of things that would've helped women to make a decision to go and give birth there. (External 2)

Despite persistent lobbying for a formal opening ceremony (the Royal College of Midwives even offered its General Secretary), none ever took place. The local media picked up on reluctance to celebrate the initiative and concluded, in the event, that the trust wanted to close the Birth Centre:

> There was a lot of media coverage about the Birth Centre, and always it was like 'The Trust are threatening to close' . . . all this kind of negative stuff in the media all the time. (Midwife 1)

Fraser *et al.* (2003) have identified media support and cooperation as essential to the success of a birth centre. The opposite happened here:

> I spent a lot of my time with journalists telling them 'Please don't print things that are negative, because you're actually undermining the Birth Centre. Although you're wanting to bring it to people's attention what the trust are doing, by doing that, you're stopping women booking.' So it's a catch-22. (External 2)

Local press coverage of possible closure led to rumours circulating, which further exacerbated the situation:

It does knock morale I think quite a bit when these rumours start going around. And of course, you see the ladies and they're hearing the rumours as well. (Midwife 7)

This negative publicity was compounded by the lack of positive publicity and marketing of the Birth Centre by the trust:

We realised we weren't getting any publicity. We didn't really have any management backing, we didn't have community midwives' backing, we had women who didn't even know about the Birth Centre. (Midwife 12)

Inevitably, the impact of this was the spiralling downwards of what was intended to be a flagship service. This will be explored in the next chapter. Moreover, the experience of the Birth Centre midwives who were working in this fragile situation was, in the main, a painful one. All of the midwives whom we interviewed had paid a personal price in their attempt to make the Birth Centre a success and provide a good service to local women despite the lack of support that they received. The Birth Centre was therefore unable to achieve its potential to be 'a place where like-minded midwives can turn the rhetoric of modern maternity care into reality, without feeling vulnerable and deviant' (Kirkham, 2003, p. 260).

REFERENCES

Ball L, Curtis P, Kirkham M. *Why Do Midwives Leave? Talking to managers.* London: Royal College of Midwives Publications; 2002.

Fraser D, Watts K, Munir F. Under the spotlight: Grantham's midwife-managed unit. In: M Kirkham (ed.) *Birth Centres: a social model for maternity care.* Oxford: Books for Midwives; 2003. pp. 39–52.

Kirkham M (ed.). *Birth Centres: a social model for maternity care.* Oxford: Books for Midwives; 2003.

Kirkham M, Morgan RK. *Why Midwives Return and their Subsequent Experience.* London: Department of Health; 2006. www.nhsemployers.org and www.rcm.org (accessed 5 December 2009).

Kirkham M, Morgan RK, Davies C. *Why Midwives Stay.* London: Department of Health; 2006. www.nhsemployers.org and www.rcm.org (accessed 5 December 2009).

Shallow H. The birth centre project. In: M Kirkham (ed.) *Birth Centres: a social model for maternity care.* Oxford: Books for Midwives; 2003. pp. 11–24.

Walsh D. *Improving Maternity Services: small is beautiful – lessons from a birth centre.* Oxford: Radcliffe Publishing Ltd; 2007.

CHAPTER 7

Spiralling downwards: interventions in the Birth Centre

INTEGRATING THE BIRTH CENTRE

The original Birth Centre midwives had, as seen earlier, been recruited from other areas. The reasons for this were summed up by two of the external people involved in the setting up of the Birth Centre:

> The midwives were intransigent to change . . . I believed it was possible to change attitude. I have become less optimistic about that. (External 1)

> The hospital midwives were not ready to take that leap because they have always worked with the doctors . . . they were just not ready to work autonomously. The community midwives were working more autonomously, but if you don't have community midwives who are promoting and supporting home births, you have to question what their skill base is then. Any midwives that worked in the Birth Centre would have to be enthusiastic; they would have to be skilled; that was essential. (External 3)

In this situation, it was logical to recruit externally, and midwives with skills and values appropriate to autonomous practice were recruited. However, they were undermined and unable to achieve the degree of clinical autonomy required for a birth centre to flourish. The midwives who had worked in the trust for longer reflected their context and its management, which was itself 'intransigent to change' in not embracing the Birth Centre.

The fact that so many of these enthusiastic midwives, recruited from elsewhere to the Birth Centre, resigned within the first year left the centre's managers with decisions to make. They could have addressed the issues that caused these midwives to leave, recruited more outside midwives, and hoped to retain them better. They could have sought to improve retention as soon as it became apparent that things were going awry, and thus not lost as many midwives as they did in that first year. Instead, they did what specifically had *not* been recommended in the feasibility study (Shallow, 2003), and they covered the vacancies by getting the existing community midwives to work shifts in the Birth Centre.

The Birth Centre represented a new way of working and an attempt to offer a family-centred approach to care. One of the managers admitted that the decision to staff the Birth Centre with community midwives was a conscious attempt to revert to a more traditional way of working:

> The model of care for the whole trust was just changing from an integrated model back to a traditional model, and changing the Birth Centre was part of that. (Manager 5)

This manager seemed generally ill at ease with the whole notion of trying to establish a separate service or develop something new or special, and she strongly felt that developments should be taken forward within the mainstream. She reveals the unease, or professional dissonance (*see* Chapter 5), that is often demonstrated by NHS managers when they are confronted with a service development that threatens to break the monolithic mould (Page, 1997; Walsh, 2007):

> It was like a separate service. To me, there didn't appear to be any buy-in from the community midwives. It was 'Oh that's the Birth Centre, that's the Birth Centre midwives, that's the Birth Centre staff', and it was completely separate . . . I think you need the leadership there definitely, but to have leadership you don't necessarily have to have a discrete set of staff . . . you need that passion and that drive in the leadership and it could be somebody rotating in and out who leads it . . . I don't think it necessarily has to be somebody who's in there all the time. (Manager 5)

This manager came into the trust after the establishment of the Birth Centre, and it seemed to us that she had been influential in the decision to integrate the community midwifery service. Many readers will doubtless question how effective leadership can be supplied by someone who is 'rotating in and out' of a post. This approach completely disregards the importance of shared philosophy and culture in practice development, as well as the different model of care within a birth centre (Shallow, 2003). These issues were to come home to roost.

STAFFING BY COMMUNITY MIDWIVES: WORKING IN AN ALIEN CULTURE

Some of the community midwives were happy to add birth centre practice to their role:

> It's been a really good experience because I've been able to get nice, normal, straightforward labours and deliveries, and it's been really nice and I've enjoyed it. (Midwife 7)

However, not all of the community midwives felt so positively about this development, as was reported by the same midwife:

> I don't think everybody is singing from the same hymnbook at the moment, and really I think it's mainly the older midwives that have found it difficult to adjust. (Midwife 7)

> It [integration with community midwifery] worked really well for some [community midwives]. Others didn't want it, that's not the way they wanted to work. They didn't want to work in the Birth Centre . . . some of them are still there and it's been a long drag for them really. (Manager 5)

Some of these midwives were clearly unprepared for their new role, and none of the managers whom we interviewed really explained why they thought that extending their role in this way, without any preparation, was appropriate. At least one manager clearly did not think that it was:

> I still remain concerned really about the midwives and how they feel about the Birth Centre, because I feel they've had a very medicalised culture. Midwives were saying to me 'Why are you wanting us to do consultant

work?'. . . Some of them really don't see our work is about practising autonomously. (Manager 3)

The insight shown by this manager indicates that at least one of the managers was aware that midwives who they themselves had identified as unsuited to birth centre practice were being asked to staff the Birth Centre, regardless of the issues that this clearly raised for the midwives, local women and the service:

> The local midwives had never had a high homebirth rate; they had never had team midwifery. . . . That's where I had involvement – going and reminding them of their personal responsibility to give women choice . . . but it's very difficult to make the horse drink even though you've taken it to water. (External 1)

Hunter (2003) and Walsh (2007) describe the skills and behaviours that support successful birth centre practice, and how these are rooted in a personal and shared value system that permeates all aspects of care and underpins safety. The failure to understand this fundamental issue had been identified very early on by the midwife who was employed on the feasibility study for this Birth Centre:

> It was painfully evident that the philosophy of care that underpins birth centre practice was being 'dumbed down' to ensure that it would be in line with uniform trust policy and procedure. . . . I could see no evidence of a commitment to birth centre principles, which are elemental to ensuring safe practice. (Shallow, 2003, p. 23)

The problems of staffing the Birth Centre with the existing community midwives were foreseen by some of the midwives who worked at the centre in the early days. Two of these midwives pointed out the clinical consequences of this strategy with regard to the transfer rate:

> They didn't do homebirths in any great numbers, so lots of those midwives were really uncomfortable about coming into the Birth Centre. . . . I said what will happen is the transfer rate will go up, the midwives will be unhappy because they feel out of their comfort zone. (Midwife 1)

> The community midwives . . . they didn't have the same philosophy that we had . . . they would transfer like that whereas we are a bit braver . . . you've got to have the same philosophy otherwise your transfer rates [go up]. (Midwife 2)

Transfer rates did rise and the number of births fell when the community midwives came to staff the Birth Centre (*see* Tables 3.1 and 3.2). Two of these midwives, who worked in the centre soon after it opened, felt that the service should have been integrated from the outset and these problems worked through while there was still the opportunity to do so, and skills rebuilt:

> I think they could have integrated the community midwives . . . from the beginning. (Midwife 1)

> I know there are some community midwives who didn't feel comfortable about home delivery let alone birth centre delivery . . . people were not using their skills and then they become less confident in their practice. . . . I felt that the Birth Centre should have been incorporated into the community. (Midwife 6)

Another midwife, representing the majority of interviewees, was opposed to integration and left when the community midwives began to work at the Birth Centre (and Birth Centre midwives also had to work in the community). She outlined what she saw as the philosophical and clinical discords that existed between the two groups of midwives:

> They said right, that's it, you're going to [integrate with] community. I thought right, that's my cue to leave, I've seen enough, I've done enough, I don't want to see or hear any more. . . . I stopped working there because I wanted to work with people who were all like-minded instead of working with a group of people that had a lot of totally different values. . . . I wanted to work with people that could do true woman-centred care and could watch and listen to labour rather than feeling for it. That's what we all had. The community midwives didn't have that . . . when I had a community midwife with me one day . . . she was fidgeting . . . and at the end she said 'I don't know how you did that . . . keeping your hands away from her.' The hardest part of midwifery is to sit on your hands and they can't, and I didn't want to work like that. (Midwife 2)

This dilution of the unified culture that had, albeit briefly, been developed among the Birth Centre midwives, and the use of community midwives to help to staff the Centre, a significant number of whom were not supportive of the birth centre concept anyway, impaired its chances of successful development. The need for enthusiasm and a common philosophy for birth centre practice was highlighted by the following external interviewee:

> If you could wave a magic wand, I would reinstate the midwives who were originally there or midwives of that calibre, promoting it . . . using it in any way possible as a centre that women can use. . . . I think it could have worked and it could have developed. (External 3)

The community midwives already had busy caseloads, and staffing shortages were soon to ensure that their working lives deteriorated as they tried to cover both their community work and their new duties at the Birth Centre. The attitude of managers to both their problems and their philosophical standpoint is clear:

> The community midwives hadn't had much involvement in the Birth Centre and really they should've been dragged kicking and screaming to have some involvement in the Birth Centre. (Manager 3)

Dragging 'kicking and screaming' midwives into birth centre practice is hardly a recipe for success in such a new venture, nor is it an enabling style of management. Given that many midwives relish the opportunity to work in a birth centre, as evidenced by the successful earlier recruitment to this one, it is unclear why reluctant midwives were asked to work in it. Some of the managers' motivation appears to have come from a desire to run a homogenous service:

> When I first came in I couldn't believe that the community midwives weren't in the Birth Centre. [At] The first opportunity, I moved the community midwives office into the Birth Centre, and there was a bit of resistance from the Birth Centre, I do have to say, to moving it in. They didn't want it in. (Manager 3)

Likewise, the Birth Centre midwives eventually had their contracts altered to integrate them into the community midwifery service. This was not the job for which they had applied and, to exacerbate matters, some of them had left community jobs to seek something new and now found themselves having to revert to jobs similar to those that they had left two years earlier:

> The writing seemed to be on the wall that, despite their successes, they were going to struggle to stay open, and the following year [2004] that became evident when the girls were told it was going to become a closed unit. They all resigned and left because they had not gone to the Birth Centre to work as a community midwife . . . they went there as birth centre midwives and they tried to develop the potential of it. (External 3)

The integration not only had adverse effects on the Birth Centre midwives, but also had serious consequences for the existing community midwives.

STAFFING BY COMMUNITY MIDWIVES: OVERLOAD, FRAGMENTATION AND BURNOUT

The decision to staff the Birth Centre with the existing, already busy, community midwives led to inevitable problems:

> Then after that they looked at an integrated service . . . but that didn't work, it fragmented community because they were doing 12-hour shifts and the community was just a mess. (Manager 1)

This manager recognised that staffing the Birth Centre over-stretched the community midwives, and that the whole project was now suspended in limbo:

> I think that the trust have got to make a decision either to close it . . . or they put the money into staffing . . . and make it work . . . it might be too late because the midwives that are left . . . have lost their motivation for it because they're absolutely tired and burnt out trying to keep it open. . . . Nobody will make a decision to support it or staff it. A big injection of money [is needed] to get community and the Birth Centre staffed properly because at the moment . . . we've got vacancies and sickness in the community and we're trying to keep the Birth Centre open. It closes more than it opens these days because we can't support the community workload. (Manager 1)

We were unable to get a clear picture of why there were financial resources to staff the Birth Centre and the community midwifery services in 2002–2003, but not subsequently. Financial pressures on the service were certainly increasing, and these seemed to serve to highlight management priorities which did not include the Birth Centre.

The cost to the community midwives of keeping the Birth Centre open was very high. It is difficult to see how a service that drained the energy of the women working in it could meet the needs of women giving birth (Deery and Kirkham, 2007). The effect on the community midwifery service was to cause fragmentation of care and staff sickness, and the Birth Centre did not function properly despite this heavy human cost.

Two of the midwives described the impact on their working and personal lives of the so-called 'integration' of the two services:

> They [the managers] just decided they would just take all the staff from the Birth Centre and put them all out on community, and each of us in turn was given the Birth Centre shifts to do. . . . You were having like a disjointed caseload . . . you were getting between six and eight on-calls a month . . . very disruptive to your own family life . . . we've lost midwives, midwives haven't been able to cope with the workload. (Midwife 11)

> We've had another midwife that's left and she wasn't replaced, so that was another four [on-calls per month to cover], so in a spate of three months that's eight on-calls between 15 of us we have to absorb . . . you don't know it's happening until a few months down the line and you think, 'Crikey, I've done six on-calls this month whereas a few months ago I was only doing four'; it creeps up on you, it really does. (Midwife 7)

This inevitably affected morale and the wider service, and further undermined the struggling Birth Centre:

> People are just like ships passing in the night, and usually it's when they're tired and you're grumbling about something and it's really not very constructive. (Midwife 7)

> I think some of them [community midwives] have become really disheartened with it [the Birth Centre], and probably feel quite shattered by the whole experience and therefore don't push it as much. (Midwife 10)

The difficulty of accessing the available support when feeling exhausted and struggling was described by the following interviewee:

> There's a supervisor there, but there again it's that grey area because you think ... it's just the fact that I've been up for 12 hours and I don't know who to call, is it important enough to wake her up at 3 o'clock in the morning and ask her what I should do? (Midwife 7)

The integration of the community midwives also aggravated the low booking figures, which were worsened by the loss of the 24-hour service. (The fall in bookings was one reason why this study was commissioned.) Some of the community midwives were reputed not to book women for the Birth Centre in an attempt to wield more control over their changing working lives:

> Some of it [poor booking numbers] may be to do with the community midwives in that they don't particularly like having to staff the Birth Centre ... certainly there was very much a difference booking wise ... some surgeries did send quite a few women and some surgeries didn't send anybody. (Midwife 8)

However, the impact on clinical care was reported to extend further than low booking numbers. One midwife felt that the number of intrapartum transfers was also being adversely affected by the exhaustion and demoralisation of the community midwives (*see* Table 3.2 for transfer figures):

> We are having a lot of transfers as well at the moment. I don't know whether it's just the midwives have lost confidence in the Birth Centre or whether it's just because they're so tired. (Midwife 11)

Another midwife recognised that rostering community midwives to work in the Birth Centre rather than having a discreet group of staff disrupted continuity and any sense of a cohesive culture:

> I would like to see staff who've really got the time and support to run it as a distinct unit ... so there's not different people coming in and out all the time. (Midwife 10)

Managers made some belated effort to ameliorate the situation by arranging a 'day out':

> We took the midwives out earlier this year for the day . . . and they spent a day together and they did some team building . . . I think that did have a positive impact initially, but I think that we're probably losing sight of that again because of the staffing issues. (Manager 3)

Attitude and culture are important in helping to build successful new maternity services, and team-building exercises, such as that commissioned here, can be very constructive. However, adverse working conditions can clearly override and negate much of their impact. Structural problems must be addressed sufficiently before cultural changes can develop, as Maslow's theory illustrates (Maslow, 1999). The manager quoted above recognised that the problems the midwives were facing started at a more basic level than attitude and culture – they lacked adequate resources.

One midwife felt that no real effort was being made to address the needs of the community midwives, and the managers were no more concerned by the loss of community midwives than they had been by their earlier failure to retain the Birth Centre midwives:

> Working in the community around my family and now . . . it will be even worse when they start working 12-hour shifts, working night shifts, doing on-calls as well . . . the number of [midwives] that couldn't cope would increase. They [managers] would prefer to watch you walk out the door. (Midwife 4)

The remedy to the situation was stated to be quite simple:

> More community midwives . . . then we can feel that we can commit to that on-call and that we don't have to worry about who's going to cover our workload next day. (Midwife 7)

In such a chronically understaffed area as maternity care (Health Commission, 2008), retention issues are crucial and this perception, whatever the actual intentions of the managers involved, is profoundly damaging to a maternity service. It is possible that retention issues will continue to be poorly addressed until they are included in the various targets that trusts have to attain. It will be ironic if 'league tables' become the route to better working conditions for midwives.

CLOSURE BY STEALTH: REDUCING CONTINUITY OF CARE

The vision for the Birth Centre was originally to provide a comprehensive local maternity service for 'low-risk' women in the area (Shallow, 2003). This initially included the Birth Centre midwives providing antenatal and postnatal care for women booking and giving birth at the Birth Centre. This attempt to provide continuity of care within the Birth Centre philosophy was an early casualty:

> We used to get to know our women, do all our own antenatals, and we used to do postnatals. . . . So they took postnatals off us and we became a glorified labour ward . . . midwifery is very intimate, this is something a lot of people don't grasp . . . it's no good having somebody come through the doors you've never met in your life before. (Midwife 2)

However, there does not appear to have been any commonality of vision for the Birth Centre. The Birth Centre midwives were attempting to follow the model described in the feasibility study (Shallow, 2003), but the trust managers do not seem to have been adhering to the same model:

> They concentrated on the number of women who gave birth at the Birth Centre and that is all; nothing else counted, childbirth preparation, antenatal checks, postnatal checks, bookings, none of that seemed to figure . . . 'You've only done that many births, therefore it's not sustainable.' (Midwife 1)

The Birth Centre's more holistic approach also led to some conflict with community midwives, who felt undermined to some degree, as the following midwife recognised:

> If we're going to give all care to this group of women . . . what does that leave the community midwives with? . . . Is there any wonder they weren't too happy about it? (Midwife 6)

These tensions and differences in approach to care do not ever seem to have been resolved, negotiated or even acknowledged by managers in order to mitigate any conflict. Instead, the two groups of midwives were increasingly thrown together and expected to find ways of working together themselves. As Birth Centre midwives became disenchanted and left, the community midwives were increasingly brought in to cover shifts as described above.

However, this further exacerbated the disintegration of any vision for the Birth Centre that had existed:

> Integrating the community midwives . . . some left at that point . . . people didn't want to work like that, they decided they would find jobs elsewhere and they did. A lot of sadness. An awful lot of sadness and despair. (External 2)

This disenchantment and loss of staff, in whom considerable investment had been made by the trust in terms of recruitment, orientation and training, seems to have been regarded as inevitable and passively accepted by managers:

> Initially it had its own midwives and now those midwives have gone . . . most of them obviously were unhappy as to the way it developed, or didn't develop. (Manager 2)

However, the loss of endeavours to increase continuity of care was only the first in a long series of steps that were taken with regard to the Birth Centre. Further compromises were soon to be initiated.

CLOSURE BY STEALTH: THE LOSS OF THE 24-HOUR SERVICE

One of the results of overstretched community staffing was the loss of 24-hour shift cover. Hallett (2003, p. 55) has argued that a move towards running a birth centre as a 'closed' service is tantamount to 'closure by stealth', and this view was shared by many of the midwives involved here. The move to staffing at night through an on-call system was strongly opposed by both the Birth Centre and the community midwives at all stages. The cessation of a full night service began with the loss of healthcare assistants at night:

> It was gradual, they sort of whittled the staff down, they didn't replace staff. On the night shift you were in the Birth Centre on your own, which was a bit unnerving, a bit scary, because it's a detached building away from other buildings. (Midwife 11)

This progressed to the Birth Centre being closed at night and serviced through an on-call rota, which was also strongly opposed. This development was seen by the Birth Centre midwives not only as unlikely to lead to any financial savings, but also as having a further detrimental effect on retention:

> I don't think it should have stopped being a 24-hour service . . . we did work it out financially, it would have been cheaper to keep it as it was, but they wanted the 'closed' option so they weren't bothered. (Midwife 12)

> So I predicted that the midwives would be unhappy and they are. I predicted that people would leave and they did. I predicted that it would cost more and I'm sure it does. (Midwife 1)

The negative implications of this type of decision, made only just over two years into the Birth Centre's existence, and during its most successful year (with 207 births), were recognised by the external individuals involved:

> To get the whole thing up and running and functioning and working had been blood, sweat and tears, and here we were in a situation where they felt it was being disassembled in essence . . . it was staving off closure by compromise. (External 3)

> My dream for that place would have been that we could have kept it open 24 hours a day. (External 1)

One midwife recognised the loss of the 24-hour shift cover as 'a nail in the coffin', and described its devastating impact on her personally:

> One day she [the secretary] came and said . . . 'You've to write to all the women and you've got to tell them that from now on' . . . it was like the first nail in our coffin . . . and I said 'Well, you can tell X that I'm not doing it . . . I'm not putting my own nails in my own coffin . . . I'm not writing to all these women to tell them . . . it's outrageous and I don't agree with it.' . . . It was round about that time I think that I'd had enough, I cried I was so upset with it all, I just cried . . . I said . . . 'I just can't fight this anymore, it's just ridiculous, it should be a flagship service, it should be the beacon.' . . . The trust should be saying 'Look what we've got and it's fantastic', and it's just this constant battle, constant battle for the staff. . . . Anyway, I did leave. (Midwife 1)

The nightly closure of the Birth Centre compromised the vision of what it was meant to be in terms of a flagship service for women. The managers involved recognised this:

> The lock-up system in itself has got all sorts of other difficulties with it . . . does the woman meet the midwife at the lock-up? . . . I mean in some ways that's quite appalling, isn't it? (Manager 2)

Waiting around in a dark car park, when in labour, for a midwife to arrive with the keys is identified as far from an ideal scenario.

CLOSURE BY STEALTH: THE CURTAILMENT OF POSTNATAL CARE

The undesirability of this situation was compounded by a decision to limit the amount of time a woman could spend in the unit after birth. This decision was linked to the loss of 24-hour staffing, as the cost of paying an on-call midwife to care for a postnatal woman into the night became a consideration. The effect of this escalating curtailment of services on women was clear to the following midwife:

> We're now told that when a woman's given birth, she's to be out of here in 5 hours. So if the baby has not established feeding . . . then they transfer them . . . it seems a bit of a shame when they've done everything here. It might be only another couple of hours but you've got this time factor. . . . I'd like to see it staffed properly and I think more people would come and use it if they thought they would be able to get a bit of postnatal support. (Midwife 9)

The transfer of a woman to the obstetric unit, located 12 miles away, for breastfeeding support is expensive and time-consuming in itself, and is disruptive to mother, baby and family. What this means in terms of providing a service is obvious to the following midwife:

> We're not offering a service . . . because half the time it's not even there [open] and I think that's frustrating for the midwives, because most of them, like me, came to work here with the expectations that it [postnatal care] would be part of our role and that was what we wanted to do. (Midwife 10)

Hallett (2003) describes the importance of providing postnatal inpatient care if birth centres are to prove successful, cost-effective and community-orientated.

CLOSURE BY STEALTH: FALLING BIRTH NUMBERS

Reinstating a 24-hour service was seen as almost impossible:

> We'd need to get about 500 through the door to staff it full-time. (Manager 3)

This is something that was unlikely to be achieved with the level of service provided, so a circular argument developed, namely that women would not use the service because its delivery was erratic and it couldn't be staffed full-time because women did not use it sufficiently. This midwife indicates how there never was an opportunity to build numbers sufficiently:

> Initially they sort of increased the numbers, they were achieving their targets, and then management decided they were going to cut the numbers of midwives down . . . then they've ended up with a situation where it's just manned Monday to Friday, 9 until 5. (Midwife 11)

The following midwife felt that the Birth Centre could have succeeded and become a popular place in which to give birth:

> In the beginning when it was staffed properly . . . demand was increasing and, if that had been left undisturbed, and nothing changed about the staff, the way it was staffed, then the numbers would have increased and increased and increased. (Midwife 11)

There is still poor understanding of the costing of maternity care (Walsh, 2007), and figures have tended to be overestimated for birth centres by comparison with obstetric units because the staff costs, which are the most measurable and quantifiable factor in maternity care costing, form a greater proportion of the total cost. Ratcliffe (2003) and McGlynn (2003) have both provided extensive evidence that the costs for birth centre births are generally lower than those for births in obstetric units. The analysis by O'Sullivan and Tyler (2007) suggests that although birth centres have a great many things to offer women and families, midwives, health trusts, and the government, financial saving is not one of them. They conclude that:

> It is highly unlikely that given current tariff levels any birth centres delivering less than 300 births a year and also not undertaking significant additional community midwifery activity for women not birthing at the unit will be financially viable. (O'Sullivan and Tyler, 2007, p. 482)

More recent work has suggested that care in birth centres may have cost benefits, but we still know little about the relationship of cost activity or numbers in birth centres and midwife-led units in comparison to obstetric care (NHS Institute for Innovation and Improvement, 2009). Hallett (2003) found that birth centres can be expensive if activity in them is low, but otherwise cost comparison is favourable. His table illustrates that cost-effectiveness for his local unit in Crowborough operates at just over 200 births per annum (Hallett, 2003, p. 56). Only once, in 2004 (its second full year of operation), did the Birth Centre in this study have more than 200 births.

The following midwife knew where she placed the blame for the decreasing birth numbers:

> It was really lack of management support; they kept pulling the rug out or adding extra bits in. (Midwife 11)

And she also knew where the solution lay:

> In an ideal world, they would staff the Birth Centre properly, they would promote it properly, they wouldn't keep pulling the rug out and changing the way they cover the Birth Centre. The women's confidence would grow in the Birth Centre, and they would feel confident that if they've booked to deliver there, they could deliver there. (Midwife 11)

The midwives were caught in the trap of having to provide and promote a service that was run in such a way that it discouraged women from using it. They could only be given the resources that they needed to provide the service if women used it, and women were not using the service because of the under-resourcing:

It'd been through this huge deluge of negativity around it that it was going to be very hard to restore confidence in women that the Birth Centre would be there when they give birth. (External 2)

The early deviations from the blueprint for the Birth Centre, which had been used to set it up (Shallow, 2003), were compounded by further decisions that went against the aspirations of the Birth Centre midwives and that undermined the working lives of the community midwives who were called to step into the breach. Although the feasibility study had proposed a single coherent vision for the Birth Centre (Shallow, 2003), this was an early casualty of the interventions by managers, who tended on the whole to adopt a short-term and pragmatic approach. In fact their decisions effectively sabotaged the Birth Centre, even if this was not their intention. This demonstrates the importance of having midwifery managers who understand the concept and ethos of birth centres (Walsh, 2007) or, more accurately, the problems that can ensue for a birth centre if midwifery managers do not possess such understanding.

REFERENCES

Deery R, Kirkham M. Drained and dumped on: the generation and accumulation of emotional toxic waste in community midwifery. In: M Kirkham (ed.) *Exploring the Dirty Side of Women's Health*. Oxford: Routledge; 2007. pp. 63–75.

Hallet R. The Crowborough birthing centre story. In: M Kirkham (ed.) *Birth Centres: a social model for maternity care*. Oxford: Books for Midwives; 2003. pp. 53–60.

Healthcare Commission. *Review of Maternity Services 2007*. London: Healthcare Commission; 2008.

Hunter M. Autonomy, clinical freedom and responsibility. In: M Kirkham (ed.) *Birth Centres: a social model for maternity care*. Oxford: Books for Midwives; 2003. pp. 239–48.

McGlynn A. Birth centres and the American spirit. In: M Kirkham (ed.) *Birth Centres: a social model for maternity care*. Oxford: Books for Midwives; 2003. pp. 191–200.

Maslow AH. *Towards a Psychology of Being*, 3rd edn. London: John Wiley & Sons; 1999.

O'Sullivan S, Tyler S. Birth centres: financially viable? *Midwives*. 2007; **10**: 481–3.

Page L. Misplaced values: in fear of excellence. *British Journal of Midwifery*. 1997: **5**: 652–4.

Ratcliffe J. The economic implications of the Edgware birth centre. In: M Kirkham (ed.) *Birth Centres: a social model for maternity care*. Oxford: Books for Midwives; 2003. pp. 131–9.

Shallow H. The birth centre project. In: M Kirkham (ed.) *Birth Centres: a social model for maternity care*. Oxford: Books for Midwives; 2003. pp. 11–24.

Walsh D. *Improving Maternity Services: small is beautiful – lessons from a birth centre*. Oxford: Radcliffe Publishing Ltd; 2007.

CHAPTER 8

The writing on the wall

DOOMED FROM THE OUTSET?

The Birth Centre underwent a rapid succession of changes in its short life, which took it ever further from the model proposed in the feasibility study and accepted by the commissioning health authority (Shallow, 2003). Each intervention exacerbated staffing problems and led to a reduced service for women. No strategic move was taken to reconstruct that service or retain its midwives, which begs the question of whether there was ever more than a short-term approach to the Birth Centre. Many of the participants in this study voiced concerns that there never was any intention within the trust to allow the Birth Centre to work or to be successful:

> I just instinctively knew that this project wasn't going to work because there was no will for it to work and the writing was on the wall. The way they wanted to harness the Birth Centre Manager in the very first instance, knowing that she wouldn't have any influence . . . I wanted to be wrong. (External 3)

> I think the way the Birth Centre had been set up, it was set up to fail because we were put midwife against midwife. (Midwife 6)

The various medical, midwifery and managerial sources of opposition to the Birth Centre have been discussed in Chapter 5. These were sufficiently powerful to seriously undermine the Birth Centre in its early days, and to have a detrimental effect on those staff who tried to make the centre a success:

> I think the rot set in even before it opened up. I think the fact that it wasn't supported by the consultants, it wasn't supported by the trust, really had a lasting effect on the midwives working in the Birth Centre. (Manager 1)

> It felt like it's been opened but the minute it's opened, there's a big question mark over its future. So I would say that instilled a sense of sadness . . . it never had an official opening because it got to a point where it was going to be stupid having an official opening for something that'd been open three years. (External 2)

This demonstrates that even a so-called 'stand-alone' birth centre is totally dependent on the structures and personnel who surround it within the wider health service (Fraser *et al.*, 2003; Hallett, 2003). The success or failure of a birth centre can only be understood in its context, and is not primarily a result of the quality or commitment of the midwives working in it.

Although the Birth Centre midwives were new to the trust and unaware of the tensions surrounding it, they quickly picked up on these as they arrived to work in their dream jobs:

> When I got there, some of the midwives said, 'Haven't they told you that we're under threat of closure all the time? Has anybody discussed it with you?' . . . And people were really worried that it hadn't been discussed with me and that I'd been misled. (Midwife 1)

This midwife, who arrived in late 2002, a few months after the Birth Centre had opened and just as the first coordinator was leaving, soon experienced at first hand the threat to the Birth Centre and how this combined with a lack of leadership to undermine the centre:

> I became more aware of how uncomfortable things were when they were talking about changing the hours and whether it was a stable service . . . and I kept saying 'We need a leader . . . we can't run an effective service without a leader.' (Midwife 1)

She describes her experience of attending meetings with managers, and demonstrates how any strategic planning that was going on even at that early stage was not focusing on building a successful birth centre:

> When we went to meetings, the conversation always was 'How can we shut it down, how can we pull out, how can we do it less?' . . . It was always kind of looking for a way of not doing it the way that we'd have loved to do it. (Midwife 1)

Kirkham (2003) sums up the impact of this kind of scenario as follows:

> Threat of closure undermines the morale of staff and service users, and can lead to a decline in bookings, which can then be used to support the argument for closure. (Kirkham, 2003, p. 258)

A POLITICAL AND FINANCIAL EXERCISE?

What is unusual here is that this began to happen so soon, almost before opening, without there having been any honeymoon period at all. Many of those who were interviewed felt that all along the whole Birth Centre project had simply been a political and financial exercise to facilitate the transfer of obstetric services to the neighbouring unit, and to yield the trust some profit from real estate:

> Then Alan Milburn made his £100 million for maternity services available, and all of a sudden, hey, there's a building over there that needs doing up, we can use that money, get it done up, open a birth centre for five years, hasn't cost us a penny. Come on, I'm not that stupid, that's exactly what they were doing . . . and I'm not the only one who's said that. (Midwife 4)

This midwife is referring to a sum of capital money that was made available by the then Health Minister, Alan Milburn. The Birth Centre, being near the town centre, was identified by a number of the interviewees as a nicely profitable investment of the money that the trust was able to procure from the 'Milburn Millions.' The Birth Centre was seen as a political sop to the local population, enabling the reconfiguration of services. The motives of the local politicians who backed it were seen as parochial and narrow by the following manager:

> They're [the Overview and Scrutiny Committee] fixated on bricks and mortar rather than what the women want. What they're fixated on is having a birthing unit in [the town], so they can have babies born in [the town]. (Manager 3)

She justified this view by describing the superficial interest taken by that powerful committee in the Birth Centre:

> They really don't understand what a birth centre is, they kept questioning us why we couldn't do epidurals there and why we couldn't have Caesarean sections there . . . really they'd not taken the time to find out anything about it. (Manager 3)

Such a political impetus behind the opening of a birth centre is not unique to this area. The birth centres in Grantham and Edgware were also at least partially driven by strong local and, in the case of the latter, national politics (Fraser *et al.*, 2003; Manero and Turner, 2003). This should work in favour of the birth centre, protecting it from the vagaries of local health managers and professional opposition. However, the lack of deeper engagement with and proper understanding of the issues suggested by the above quoted extract may explain why the political support in this instance did not help the Birth Centre as much as it might have done. Another manager echoes this pervasive sense that the Birth Centre was a means to an end, rather than an end in itself:

> Originally it felt like a token gesture . . . I think it was set up as a token gesture. (Manager 4)

The same manager also suggests that it was never seen as a long-term enterprise:

> It might have been open about a year, there were rumblings even then that it would be closing. (Manager 4)

These words are echoed by another managerial colleague:

> There was some doubt about whether the Birth Centre would even stay open, you know there's always been this cloud over it: is it going to close, isn't it going to close? (Manager 5)

They are also echoed, more strongly, by some of the midwives:

> When we were first in post . . . we were told quite categorically the Birth
> Centre was only a five-year plan . . . all I got was a pack of lies, absolute pack
> of lies . . . the porters would . . . say 'It's only going to be here for two years' –
> this is all we got all the time – rumour, rumour, rumour, and nobody would
> dispel them for us, not that we believed them anyway, I got to a point in the
> end where I believed nobody. (Midwife 2)

> I started to have feelings that the people had never been entirely honest with
> me, and one of the first meetings I went to, I suddenly found out that the
> Birth Centre had a lifespan of five years. (Midwife 6)

When interviewing senior managers and key external players, we could find
no evidence that this rumour of a planned five-year lifespan had any truth
to it. However, the consistency of perception that the Birth Centre had no
long-term future does not seem to have been clearly contradicted in either
words or actions by the trust. These quoted extracts and the situation that
gave rise to them may imply that the managers felt that any effort on their
part to make the Birth Centre a success would have been misplaced and
futile, and may explain the contradictory position they took, described in
Chapter 5. They also show the extent of the uncertainty under which the
midwives were labouring.

THE IMPACT OF CONSTANT CHANGE OF SENIOR MANAGERS

Other difficulties that the managers faced included the ever-changing
management tiers above them in the trust, and its constrained financial
circumstances. This meant not only a lack of focus on the Birth Centre by
those with power, but also a need to repeat previous briefings on a regular
basis:

> The trust had always been financially encompassed, they were always in the
> red . . . and, of course, merging of trusts. (Manager 4)

> We've had two chief execs in four years and everyone had a different take on it
> . . . under extreme financial pressure as the trust is, that impacts on the Birth
> Centre as well. . . . We've got a new chief exec come in so it's my opportunity

to lobby him, this'll be the third, it's a whole new world when you get a new chief exec. (Manager 3)

The lack of continuity of managers at the top level of the trust was recognised as a factor by the Birth Centre midwives as well. One midwife described how the fast rate of turnover of senior trust managers constrained long-term strategic planning and consistency of approach:

> So you just feel that the people that make these decisions can make them because they're going after they make them. There's no permanence in the service and the people who are running the service. The only permanence is in the people who are delivering the service at the end of the line. And now . . . with all that's hanging over us, you don't know if there's going to be any permanence there. (Midwife 11)

One of the managers gave an example of this lack of continuity and consistency arising from the rapid turnover of senior management staff, and the negative impact of this on the Birth Centre:

> There is one director who says the Birth Centre will not shut, and I said, 'That's great and I'm pleased you said that, but on the other hand you've got to commit posts' . . . I know we need these two posts, I thought I'd got it all signed and sealed, and then one of the other directors threw their spoke in and said no. (Manager 3)

Lack of continuity of personnel at *all* levels was seen as having an exacerbating effect and as having led directly to many of the problems that were encountered:

> It's had that much change at the top, change of midwives . . . are the community midwives really selling it as they should . . . how many of the community midwives are actually committed to it, you know, because they had it thrust upon them? (Manager 2)

The state of constant flux in the broader health service is clearly having a serious impact on effective service delivery at grass-roots level, and causing dysfunction at middle management level:

> I've no idea [what the outcome will be], no idea to be honest . . . a new chief
> exec . . . the trust financial position . . . the health economy is in such flux,
> PCTs all being reconfigured, mega financial pressures, the SHA [strategic
> health authority] chain being reconfigured, the place is in turmoil . . . and
> I think we'll stand still. (Manager 3)

This culture of rapid change in more senior NHS managerial posts is
clearly detrimental in a situation such as this. Change becomes nothing
more than turmoil and uncertainty, lacking any strategic input or element
of consistent development. Accountability becomes a temporary and
tradable irrelevance as long-term commitment to developments becomes
more rare. This is a broader issue for the NHS, but the way in which this
managerial culture of 'moving on' affects services is illustrated well in this
instance.

THE POLITICAL IMPEDIMENTS TO CLOSURE: PAWNS IN A GAME

The lack of strategic drive to keep the Birth Centre open or to help it to flourish begs the question of why it had not closed at the time of our interviews
(late 2006). The participants had a fairly consistent answer to this, which
was that they felt it was kept open by default, as it was politically impossible
to be seen to close it:

> What's keeping it open? Political . . . there's pressure from the Overview and
> Scrutiny Committee. (Manager 3)

> Most of us feel that management can't close it because it's too much of a
> political issue to close it. . . . We don't want to close it, we want to staff it in
> a way that's going to work for us and for the clients. (Midwife 11)

It was pointed out that although the trust claimed it supported the Birth
Centre, its actions, specifically in terms of financial support, belied that
claim of support. This made life particularly difficult for those involved in
front-line management of the Birth Centre:

> The trust say 'We want it to stay open', politicians say 'We want it to stay
> open', and the women say they want it to stay open, but here we are trying
> to manage this service which isn't functioning as well as it could. So I think

that people sort of need to put their money where their mouths are . . . if they want the service, then they are going to have to fund it. (Manager 3)

The issue of finances will be discussed more fully later in this chapter.

One of the managers pointed out the difficulty of closing the unit in the face of recent Department of Health rhetoric regarding the importance of choice:

> Has it had a reprieve because of all the government initiatives coming through? . . . If they close it, it's going against all what they're saying, isn't it? Like women's choice and everything? (Manager 2)

The political difficulties facing the trust in closing the Birth Centre were seen as only a temporary impediment to closure. Many of the participants were of the opinion that a way would be found to close the unit which would involve manipulation of the midwives by making their working lives increasingly impossible, and indeed during the writing of this book the Birth Centre closed. The participants, especially the midwives, felt that they were pawns in a game that was being played out by people above them in the NHS hierarchy:

> Ever since before I'd arrived, they've been 'It's going to close . . . it's just a matter of time' . . . and when we've said, 'Look, what's going on? What is happening?' we've always had 'Oh no, we want to keep it open' . . . but then what actually happens seems to contradict that. . . . Ultimately we expect the decision will be made to close it, and I think that's something we feel the management is working towards, but almost by the back door because, although they can't justify shutting it, they'll run it into the ground and say it's not functioning . . . we could keep it open in the night if we were all willing to do eight, nine, ten on-calls a month, but there comes a point where you . . . can't do that permanently . . . they're almost forcing your hand to pull back and say 'Well, it's not viable.' (Midwife 10)

In other words, the midwives would be forced to do what no one else had the courage to do – close the Birth Centre. This idea that the midwives themselves would eventually be cornered into acquiescing to the closure of the service was echoed by a number of the participants:

It's just the uncertainty for the women . . . the fact that we feel overworked and we also feel that management would quite like it if we stood up and said 'We can't cover, we can't do this anymore', because then they can blame us for the decision, rather than it coming from them or some official source. We feel they're sort of chipping away and not really supporting us so that in the end we can say 'We can't do this any longer' and they've got their excuse then to close down. (Midwife 11)

That's what they do, close it by stealth, because what they do is make it impossible for you to manage and then you have to say 'Well, actually we can't do this' . . . we lost three members of staff and none of them were replaced . . . which we carried for quite a long time doing 'extras' . . . it wasn't safe at all . . . and they were saying 'Look, you're not managing, you can't do it, it's driving you into the ground, you're working all hours.' Well, yes, because you've never replaced [the midwives] who've left, we haven't got a team leader, we spend all our days off at meetings trying to keep the Birth Centre afloat. (Midwife 1)

It appeared that this strategy, if it was a strategy, was beginning to bear fruit even at the time when the interviews took place:

There are a few midwives that I've heard say they wouldn't mind if it shut, really because of the on-call commitment . . . every single time you're first on call, and you're called out for a long time, and you're tired, and that's when it has a knock-on effect of you not liking it. (Midwife 7)

One midwife stated that the original ethos of the Birth Centre had been so compromised that there was no point in expending further energy on it. The Birth Centre was not achieving the vision that had been set out for it in her view, and her solution was radical:

If it's going to close, let's close it, let's get on and . . . basically focus on home births . . . we can offer that service at home. You don't need the building to come into . . . she [manager] wants us all to look the same, she wants us to look clinical so we look like professional people. The Birth Centre midwives didn't wear uniform . . . I just can't see why we need to be in a building with a uniform on. (Midwife 4)

Again the importance of uniform as a symbol of conflicting philosophies of midwifery and models of care is apparent (*see* Chapters 4 and 9). In the end, and whatever the difficulties, closure was seen by many of the midwives as inevitable:

> They're wanting to close it and they haven't been allowed to, so they'll find a way. I don't think they'll recruit [to vacancies]. Am I being very sceptical? They don't want it, the trust, the obstetricians, they don't want it. (Midwife 6)

> To close it by strikes, failing to achieve . . . and they can say 'Well, nobody's using the Birth Centre, so obviously there's no reason to have the Birth Centre here, so let's close you.' (Midwife 12)

However, the Birth Centre continued to limp on, having only 61 births in 2007, and finally closing at the end of that year, after our data collection. The closure, when it did occur, was probably a relief to the overstretched staff who were working in its then very limited service. The fact that it managed to survive for so long is a testament to the dedication of the midwives who carried on refusing to give in to the manipulation that they identified in the above quoted extracts.

'A LUXURY WE CAN'T AFFORD': THE FINANCING AND UNDER-FINANCING OF THE BIRTH CENTRE

As described earlier, the Birth Centre was purchased with what became known as the 'Milburn millions.' It was decorated and furnished to a reasonably high level at the time of opening. However, by the time of these interviews, some five years later, it was in need of redecoration and some repair (for example, the roof had leaked, causing some damp patches in one of the rooms). The midwives felt that there was no prospect of any work being done on the Birth Centre, and regarded this as another indicator of a desire to close it.

The managers had quite a lot to say about the funding of the Birth Centre, and explained many of the actions described earlier in this chapter as arising from financial constraints. They stated that the Birth Centre was inadequately funded. In part, this was felt to be because although it was actually a more expensive service than mainstream maternity care, there was no allowance made for or validation of this fact:

> Philosophically they [the trust] didn't particularly agree with it. Another thing is they had to recognise the Birth Centre is not a cheap service, but if you're gonna do this, you should do it properly, and you should resource it properly, and there's never been that recognition or that firing up to it. (Manager 3)

This is an important point, and it relates to an earlier one about the monolithic tendencies of NHS maternity care, discussed in Chapter 4. The idea that services should aim for financial parity if they are to be equitable, a notion that is prevalent in the NHS, puts any service development such as this at an immediate disadvantage:

> It was always under the spotlight for financial reasons, trying to take money out. (Manager 3)

One-to-one schemes and team midwifery have fallen foul of similar impulses to maintain financial parity across all types of service delivery (Page, 1997). If one form of care delivery costs more than another, it is seen as untenable, or even inequitable. This has serious implications for birth centres, but is not addressed by Department of Health promotions of birth centres (Shribman, 2007). More recently, financial savings have been put forward as a rationale for increasing the normal birth rate (NHS Institute for Innovation and Improvement, 2006). Whatever the merits of a financial argument as opposed to a health argument for normal birth may be, the implications that this has for the UK's birth centres are as yet uncertain.

In recent years the maternity services have seen a cut in their share of the NHS financial cake from 3% to 2% (Cohen, 2008). This, combined with a rise in the birth rate (Cohen, 2008), and the requirement for trusts to 'balance the books', has put maternity care under considerable strain, as outlined by the following interviewee:

> There's no doubt in my mind why midwives are leaving, because they're being expected to hold ever higher caseloads, do more and more and more, and their time is so limited that to expect midwives to do more on-call [for the Birth Centre], I don't see that happening at the moment because of the constraints on the service . . . and the financial cutbacks, so it will be seen as a luxury we can't afford, and that's a great shame . . . because women are suffering in the acute services. (External 3)

> It's balancing the books . . . they had that money there once and what's different, what's changed, where's that money gone to? (Midwife 11)

Some of the anxiety about finances was attributed to a fear of litigation – the ghost at the banquet of any discussion of maternity services development:

> I think people were worried that things would go wrong and litigations, from the trust point of view . . . it was always 'What if this goes wrong or if that goes wrong?' (Manager 4)

It is hard to quantify just how much of a role, if any, a fear of litigation has played in the history of the Birth Centre. There is no evidence that birth centres are any less safe than large maternity units in terms of outcomes (Porter and Tinsley, 2003). The Birth Centre had no seriously adverse incidents or, in today's healthcare parlance, 'serious untoward incidents' (SUIs). The steps taken by managers in terms of reducing staffing of the Birth Centre, running it from an on-call system at night, and curtailing the length of postnatal stay, could all have added to potential 'risk' rather than reducing it, so it seems unlikely that the unit or its midwives were ever seriously considered unsafe.

The correctly predicted closure of the Birth Centre and the many changes that were implemented prior to its closure were seen as primarily financially driven and largely inexorable:

> If they've got money shortages, the one thing that'll go will be the Birth Centre . . . the fact that women are now being kicked out four hours after giving birth, to me, is absolutely atrocious. (Midwife 12)

However, this did not stop some of the midwives from continuing to do their utmost to keep the Birth Centre open right up until the end:

> There's a lot of things that are trying to get off the ground at the moment to expand the role of the Birth Centre, because . . . that's the only way we're going to stay open, if we can show that it can be more useful than just delivering babies. (Midwife 7)

The odds were stacked against them. To reverse the long story of the dismantling of the Birth Centre which has been outlined in this chapter would always take more than anything the midwives could do by themselves. We had hoped that they would succeed, and that local women would eventually have a birth centre that offered a full and sustained service along the lines originally envisaged (Shallow, 2003). However, the sorry story of the Birth Centre was summarised as follows by one of the managers:

> I think the Birth Centre's had a really, really chequered history . . . and I feel sad about it really in a lot of ways. (Manager 3)

REFERENCES

Cohen H. NHS maternity services. Early Day Motion 1112. In: *Hansard*, UK Parliament, 4 March 2008.

Fraser D, Watts K, Munir F. Under the spotlight: Grantham's midwife-managed unit. In: M Kirkham (ed.) *Birth Centres: a social model for maternity care*. Oxford: Books for Midwives; 2003. pp. 39–52.

Hallet R. The Crowborough birthing centre story. In: M Kirkham (ed.) *Birth Centres: a social model for maternity care*. Oxford: Books for Midwives; 2003. pp. 53–60.

Kirkham M (ed.). *Birth Centres: a social model for maternity care*. Oxford: Books for Midwives; 2003.

Manero E, Turner L. Users in the driving seat. In: M Kirkham (ed.) *Birth Centres: a social model for maternity care*. Oxford: Books for Midwives; 2003. pp. 63–70.

NHS Institute for Innovation and Improvement. *Delivering Quality and Value: focus on normal birth and reducing Caesarean section rates*. Coventry: NHS Institute for Innovation and Improvement; 2006.

Page L. Misplaced values: in fear of excellence. *British Journal of Midwifery*. 1997; 5: 652–4.

Porter R, Tinsley V. The Wiltshire model. In: M Kirkham (ed.) *Birth Centres: a social model for maternity care*. Oxford: Books for Midwives; 2003. pp. 25–38.

Shallow H. The birth centre project. In: M Kirkham (ed.) *Birth Centres: a social model for maternity care*. Oxford: Books for Midwives; 2003. pp. 11–24.

Shribman S. *Making it Better: for mother and baby*. London: Department of Health; 2007.

CHAPTER 9

The Birth Centre: ideals, models and tensions

THE IDEAL SERVICE: THE MIDWIVES' VISION

The 13 midwives from the Birth Centre whom we interviewed were asked to describe what their ideal maternity service would look like. Their responses are summarised in Table 9.1.

TABLE 9.1 The Birth Centre ideals, models and tensions

Characteristics of ideal maternity service	Number of respondents
More/real choice for women	9
Midwife-led care	8
More midwives	7
The Birth Centre	7
Continuity of care from booking to postnatal/NHS Midwifery Model/ caseload midwifery/team midwifery	7
Home birth	3
Better birth environments and facilities	3
Independent midwifery	2
More local obstetric services/less distance to obstetric services	2
Woman-led care	1
Family-centred care	1

Choice for women and the need for more midwives were seen as being closely interlinked. Lack of true choice was perceived as a direct consequence of staff shortages, and these two issues were regarded as crucial by most of the midwives who were interviewed. The midwives felt that women were being 'conned' into thinking that they had choices when those choices were either illusionary or constrained by the shortage of midwives. Many were scornful or dismissive of the whole choice agenda, believing that women are not offered any choice worthy of the name in the maternity services at present.

Many respondents felt that the Birth Centre was still close to an ideal service, despite its problems:

> You should only go to hospital if you need hospital service. I think if you don't you should have your baby at home or in a birth centre. I think women should only be in hospital when they need to be. I think that rather than earn your right to be at home, you ought to earn your right to be in hospital. (Midwife 1)

However, one of the managers felt that there were good reasons why women may not prefer a free-standing birth centre at some distance from an obstetric unit:

> I think the women's preferred option would be a midwife-led unit next to a delivery suite, because that's something else that puts the women off – the fact that if there's a problem they've got to get in an ambulance and go 10 miles to the consultant unit. . . . I think women would choose to deliver there [the Birth Centre] more if the distances weren't so great. (Manager 1)

The opinion expressed above has a professional ring to it, although it was put forward as 'women's preferred option.' This view was not expressed by women who had used this Birth Centre or that studied by Walsh (2007). Continuity of care was mentioned in various guises as fundamental to ideal midwifery care, including the NHS Midwifery Model (van der Kooy, 2006), the New Zealand model (Pairman and Guilliland, 2003), caseloading and independent midwifery. There was considerable criticism of the current state of the maternity services in the UK:

> I think maternity care in this country is absolute rubbish, you know: I think a whole load needs to be done and I don't know what the answer is. Well,

> I do, it's the independent midwives' community midwifery model.' [see www.independentmidwives.org.uk] (Midwife 2)

Some of the midwives felt that home birth was the ideal, and that birth centres and home births were similar in many ways:

> I always personally preferred home births, and I have got mixed views about birth centres, because I think . . . 'Why do you want to come into a building to give birth when you can get the same service at home?' (Midwife 4)

> There isn't a jot of difference to having your baby at the Birth Centre and having your baby at home . . . people do find it difficult to understand why somebody would choose a birth centre, but everybody has their reasons, it might just be that the walls are thin and they don't want their neighbours to hear or that they don't want the mess. (Midwife 1)

The issues raised here are interesting. There is clearly a lot of truth in the assertion that birth centre birth and home birth are very similarly positioned in relation to mainstream care. Matters of transfer and emergency care, which are the issues of safety that are of prime consideration, have to be addressed in broadly similar ways whether at home or in a birth centre. For midwives the concerns are the same, namely how emergencies will be dealt with and whether transfer can be effected quickly if the need arises.

WHY BIRTH CENTRES?

Midwife 4 asks a pertinent question. What is the point of birth centres? What do they offer over and above a good homebirth service? Midwife 1 suggests some answers (thin walls, and the mess involved), but these are only a partial explanation, especially in relation to the financial investment in birth centres. Manager 3 recognises that birth centres may require greater investment in midwifery time, too:

> It is exactly the same as having a home confinement, really. . . . Unless you're getting the numbers through, it's very inefficient in midwife time compared to a home confinement, 'cos with a home confinement you can go, can't you, deliver the woman and you can be out of the house in an hour, can't you. (Manager 3)

Understanding the purpose of birth centres is fundamental, and without this understanding of their role and their potential as effective and efficacious birth institutions, birth centres will continue to be favoured or threatened according to the limited personal, financial or political perspectives of those in charge of them. Understanding their role is crucial if they are to become a fully integrated part of maternity care.

Kirkham (2003) has outlined some of the underlying purpose and meaning of birth centres. They offer a community and geographical locus and focus for the rite of passage of birth, bringing together women, midwives and the community in a public and clean, but private and homely place. Birth centres help to build a common culture of nurture or 'pampering' and midwifery skill to aid physiological birth and the transition to mothering (Kirkham, 2003; Walsh, 2007). This makes them more than a mirror image of home birth. Birth centres represent or offer:

➤ choice
➤ location of birth within a community or geographical area
➤ homebirth-like facilities for women who are homeless or who have poor housing
➤ inclusion and welcoming of partners and family into the birth environment
➤ a place of safety and retreat from daily life
➤ a community hub
➤ a valuing of social outcomes from maternity care.

Boulton *et al.* (2003) have listed the following reasons why women choose a birth centre over home birth:

➤ the availability of facilities such as pools and birth stools
➤ having a midwife present at all times
➤ less mess
➤ home life and children not disrupted
➤ a break from domestic responsibilities
➤ cleanliness and tidiness.

The purpose and value of birth centres are therefore more cultural and social than medical, and they help women and midwives to share experience and meaning as well as physical space.

A SOCIAL MODEL FOR MATERNITY CARE

Birth centres have been described as providing a social model for maternity care (Kirkham, 2003), where the woman is seen as able to birth her baby with support from those close to her and from her midwife. Relationships are central to this model, and every effort is made to foster trusting, enduring, equal relationships between the woman and her peers and her midwife. This is a partnership model that minimises power differences, develops women's strength, and is experienced as mutually enabling for mother and midwife. This model emphasises the need for the woman to feel safe, thus promoting the production of the childbearing hormone oxytocin, which is essential for labour and breastfeeding. This is very different from the medical model, with its emphasis on expert knowledge and technology, and the power of the obstetrician to rescue the woman and her baby from the defects of her body. This can devalue women's knowledge and strength and leave them feeling fearful, which increases the production of adrenaline, an oxytocin antagonist. Clearly women need choice, and different models suit different people and different circumstances.

A social model and its potential were clearly stated in the feasibility study for this Birth Centre (Shallow, 2003), and were espoused as a philosophy by those in the health authority who originally commissioned the Birth Centre, and by the midwives who initially came to work there. However, there is very little evidence that this model was valued or even acknowledged by management at any level within the trust. Many of the problems of the Birth Centre could be seen as originating from management attempts to enforce one model of care across all of the maternity services locally, as symbolised by the issue of uniforms (see below).

We could find no evidence of attempts to foster the collegiality and interdisciplinary support that are seen as so important in establishing and providing role models for a social model of maternity care (Brodie and Leap, 2008). Inter-professional collaboration and trust are regarded as essential for developing a social model of maternity care, promoting physiological birth and improving services (Brodie and Leap, 2008; Homer *et al.*, 2008; Page, 2008). However, no one in this study saw it as their role to facilitate the development of such trust and collaboration between professionals. Indeed many of the events relating to the Birth Centre demonstrated a lack of collaboration and served to undermine trust (*see* Chapters 5 and 6). The Birth Centre midwives themselves had little power to develop the social model of birth at any wider level than their relationships with individual mothers. When their antenatal role was removed and the opening hours of the Birth Centre were restricted, even this central relationship was threatened. This threat to relationships was not acknowledged by management when these cuts in service were instituted. Indeed it may be argued that these relationships were curtailed because they were seen as 'elitist' and deviant from the medical model, rather than as representing a very different social midwifery model which could, with mutual benefit, exist alongside the medical model.

PLACE AND TERRITORY

The physical setting is important, as it can help to reinforce the 'specialness' of the rite of passage of birth and the care of women undertaking this. It can help women to feel safe at a very vulnerable time. Women who visited the Birth Centre responded to its homely environment, and this often prompted them to choose to give birth there:

> Most women are really enthusiastic, but some women were very definitely 'Oh, I couldn't do that, it's not my thing', and other women are sort of in the middle ground and will come and have a look. And to be honest, if they are middle ground, when they come to look, most of them end up coming [to give birth here]. (Midwife 10)

The physical ambience of a birth centre is therefore important. Walsh (2007) has discussed this extensively with regard to the decoration and maintenance of the birth centre that he studied, and he links it to the idea of 'nesting' (Walsh, 2007, p. 46). Boulton *et al.* (2003) found that environment was important to women using their local birth centre (in Edgware). The importance of environment was recognised by the midwives who worked in the Birth Centre that is the subject of this study:

> I think it's lovely. I think as a building it's been done really nicely, and also the concept behind it and sort of the philosophy behind it, which is really part of what encouraged me to apply for a job in the first place. (Midwife 10)

Midwifery managers also showed awareness that a special environment for birth was integral to the birth centre concept:

> I know a lot of people have actually said that there was too much money spent on the Birth Centre, but I mean if you're doing something, it's got to be done right. (Manager 2)

Beyond the physical space, the Birth Centre midwives succeeded in creating 'birth territory' (Fahy et al., 2008, p. 12) where women felt safe and able to give birth. The early statistics verify this, as do the views of service users.

However, the midwives themselves did not feel safe and able to fully use their skills in the birth territory of which they sought to be the 'guardians' (Fahy et al., 2008). They lacked autonomy and were unsuccessfully *'fighting really to be left alone, for them to leave us how we were working'* (Midwife 1). They felt powerless and frustrated (*see* Chapter 6). Just when the Birth Centre's birth rate was showing a healthy increase, the midwives' 24-hour presence in the centre was threatened. This left the Birth Centre midwives in a very difficult position. Birth centres have long been established as midwives' territory (Kirkham, 1987, 2003), where they feel secure, to which they are committed (Walsh, 2007), and which provide a safe base within which they can exercise their clinical skills. The midwives in this study were not able to establish their territory. It is difficult for midwives to facilitate safety and empowerment for women if they are feeling threatened and undermined in their work setting.

THE SOCIAL ROLE OF THE BIRTH CENTRE

The Birth Centre did not live up to all expectations, particularly with regard to the ideal of birth centres as 'community hubs':

> I was very disappointed when I first saw the building . . . I expected it to be a building where people could meet, when they thought 'I need to breastfeed, oh let's go to the Birth Centre' . . . I suppose a bit like what the Children's Centres are trying to encompass. (Midwife 4)

It is difficult for employees of an NHS trust that is focused on acute hospital-based care to achieve such a community focus. Nevertheless, the literature suggests that a social model of maternity care needs to be rooted in its community:

> We suggest that midwives are only able to facilitate a social model of birth if they [re]claim a style of working that is both physically and philosophically based in the community. It is ultimately questionable whether midwifery can flourish within the hegemony of fragmented hospital systems that stifle the ability to practise 'woman-centred care' in a way that enriches the potential for women, and therefore their families and communities, to be more powerful. (Brodie and Leap, 2008, p. 157)

The low level of home births locally suggests that although the community midwives were working in their community, they lacked such philosophical grounding.

This community-centred aspect of birth centre practice was not mentioned in the 'ideal service' descriptions of the midwives, and may have left them vulnerable to criticism by their many detractors. One manager made the following interesting comment:

> The community midwives expected the Birth Centre to be run as a community service. . . . I expected there to be drop-ins, parentcraft sessions, breastfeeding support, more of a community facility, but the core midwives ran it as a mini-hospital. They ran it as a delivery suite with an elitist antenatal and postnatal service. (Manager 1)

This interesting comment, whether justified or not, demonstrates that other notions of an 'ideal service' were and are current. The constraints on developing the full potential of this Birth Centre from the outset have been described elsewhere (Shallow, 2003). However, it is clear from this study that opportunities for building a mutually shared vision or ideal once the Birth Centre had been opened were not taken. The 'ideal service' dialogue that occurred to some extent during the planning stage (Shallow, 2003) seems to have been quickly superseded by preoccupation with, metaphorically speaking, choice of sticking plaster with regard to the cracks that inevitably appeared, as discussed elsewhere in this work.

It is interesting that in the recent study published as *Birth Models that Work* (Davis-Floyd *et al.*, 2009), one of only two examples from the UK is a birth centre (Walsh, 2009). This long established birth centre acted as a focus for 'rejection of assembly-line birth' (Walsh, 2009, p. 165) and 'resisting bureaucracy' (Walsh, 2009, p. 168). The midwives there and in other birth centres we know had developed a way of assisting birth that is flexible, trusting, respectful, democratic and sustainable. The network of reciprocal relationships and the common values in such a model are seen as enhancing social capital for the local community and the individuals concerned. Such achievements are rarely seen in relation to birth, and are more familiar in relation to community health and development endeavours. The benefits of 'a common ideology that birth is normal and that women are its protagonists' (Davis-Floyd *et al.*, 2009, p. 442) are personally and socially far reaching. Sadly, in the birth centre that we studied they were not allowed to develop.

UNIFORMS: A SYMBOL OF THE TENSIONS RELATING TO THE BIRTH CENTRE

One of the midwives mentioned 'no uniforms' as being part of her ideal service. The issue of uniforms arose several times during the interviews in different contexts, and has been mentioned elsewhere in this study. The importance of uniform or rather 'no uniforms' seems to be intrinsic to many of the midwives' visions and aspirations.

Conversely, uniforms were seen as emblematic of the tensions between different models of care and concepts of midwifery:

> The Director of Nursing . . . took umbrage at the fact that we were not wearing uniform and hadn't asked – my god we are only adults after all (can you tell I am very bitter?) – so we had to go back into uniforms . . . how pathetic, so pedantic, so petty, absolutely petty they were. (Midwife 2)

Clearly uniform represents something important, not only for the midwives but also for the manager who insisted on it. Although the midwives at the Birth Centre did stop wearing uniform again for a while, the midwives who were working there at the time when the interviews were conducted were wearing uniform again.

Uniform represents conformity (Flint, 1995). It marks the wearer out as one of a group, as belonging to or loyal to an organisation or institution, and it represents a subsuming of the individual or personal in a collective mission. It also sets the wearer apart from the general population and emphasises one aspect of their being over all others. Thus the individual becomes a nurse, a scout, a schoolgirl, or a soldier, for example, and this role is emphasised over and above that of the individual personality:

> She [the manager] wants us to all look the same, she wants us to look clinical so we look like professional people. The Birth Centre midwives didn't wear uniform until they were asked to change when the Birth Centre and community [midwifery service] got back together. I just can't see why we need to be in a building with uniform on. (Midwife 4)

'New midwifery' (Page, 2000) emphasises relational, personal and individual aspects of care. This social model of midwifery demands that midwives face outward from their employing organisations and form personal alliances and relationships with the women and families whom they serve. Individualised care cuts both ways, as understanding a woman as an individual, and building a relationship of trust and support with her, can only be predicated upon offering oneself to some extent as an individual personality to her. The idea of 'knowing one's midwife' involves more than just having that midwife's name and contact number. Our choice of clothes is one way of helping others to know and recognise us, and it conveys messages about us that others can interpret:

> I used to think uniform didn't matter, but now I think it does. It gives the wrong messages. (Midwife 13)

> We're talking about a home [type] environment, so for me that means sort of casual [clothing], not specific nursing or midwife uniforms. 'No, they have to wear uniforms.' . . . I got quite involved with that and then we said 'OK, we'll have some sort of dress code' but, you know, that still defeats the object if you're trying to put a woman at ease. . . . I think, on the whole, ordinary clothes in that particular setting would have been fine . . . it seemed as though 'OK we can facilitate that', but then I know, a few months after I left, it came back as completely uniforms. (Midwife 6)

The fact that this issue proved so obdurate suggests that it represents the crux of the tensions between opposing models of care and midwifery ideals. Uniforms and what they represent need to be carefully considered when developing services, and not dismissed as a minor or inconsequential detail. The midwives in this study recognised the importance of uniform as a symbol of the conflicts in which they were caught up, and the failure to recognise that birth centre care was a different model of care from that practised in a consultant unit.

There seems to be a resonance between what women and midwives want from maternity services. In terms of the range of services, the environment in which these are offered, the purpose of these services, the culture of birth, the emphasis of care, the importance of relationships and the social nature of birth, the needs and desires of women and of midwives are parallel. The midwives whom we interviewed had briefly come close to creating their ideal service, and research conducted with local women (reference has been withheld to maintain anonymity) shows that they succeeded in delivering what women want, too. It is unfortunate that the ideal could not be sustained and that it was achieved at such a high personal cost to so many of the midwives whom we interviewed.

POWER, AUTHORITY AND MANAGEMENT

The Birth Centre was established at the instigation of the health authority, not of the trust which was required to run it. The members of the health authority who had instigated the plan soon moved to other areas. It was therefore of crucial importance that there was an advocate for the Birth Centre who had easy access to senior trust management. This key voice was lacking. The Birth Centre coordinator was of a grade that did not give her access to senior management and its planning processes – a problem that was forecast in the feasibility study. The lack of an authoritative link with senior management constrained the autonomy of the Birth Centre midwives and prevented them from fulfilling all the potential of their role.

None of the midwifery managers were energetic advocates for the Birth Centre, as it was an additional area of responsibility that they had not chosen. No one with management authority in the trust identified the Birth Centre as their project or as one worthy of their energetic support. As it was no one's priority within trust management, the Birth Centre languished due to lack of funding, management and publicity.

This lack of an authoritative advocate for the Birth Centre who had access to management differentiates this Birth Centre from many others which were successful, such as the Edgware Birth Centre. In the early days of the Edgware Birth Centre, the supervisor of midwives played a key role in building midwives' clinical skills, confidence and autonomy. One of the ways in which this was achieved was through her facilitating the midwives in their development of clinical guidelines for the birth centre:

> It was considered important that midwives should be able to decide what guidelines they should use and be actively involved in the development and implementation of these guidelines. To enable them in this activity they needed to understand the theory underpinning the design and use of guidelines. Whilst they were encouraged to undertake the work themselves, the supervisor was available to give advice on the process. (Jones, 2000, p. 156)

The supervisor of midwives at Edgware also facilitated group reflection on practice, which served to test and further develop the guidelines. These supervisory activities were experienced as empowering by the birth centre midwives. The supervisor there also saw it as part of her role to identify and endeavour to deal with resistance to the Edgware Birth Centre in its early days. The interpretation of supervision at the Birth Centre that we studied was very different, with no perceived need for guidelines specific to, or owned by, the Birth Centre. It is noteworthy that the additional training that was received by the newly recruited midwives before the Birth Centre opened took place within the consultant unit, not in the Birth Centre or specifically related to the practice and philosophy of the latter. Enhancing the clinical autonomy of these midwives was not an aim for supervisors or management.

Midwifery autonomy can be seen as an important issue here. Lack of autonomy to achieve what they see as good practice is one of the reasons why midwives leave the profession in England (Ball *et al.*, 2002). Lack of autonomy is also consistent with working to an 'economies of performance' model (Stronach *et al.*, 2002), where clinical work depends on midwives becoming obedient technicians in order to sustain working within bureaucratic structures and imperatives (Deery, 2010; Deery and Fisher, 2010; Deery and Hunter, 2010).

Alternatively, 'ecologies of practice' develop when midwives are facilitated to draw upon a wealth of diverse knowledge, experience and influences, including relational and experiential knowledge developed in their private lives and in the communities in which they live. However, when clinical work is overly determined by managerialist practices, holistic and authentic forms of care, such as birth centre work, can become stifled (Deery and Fisher, 2010). Therefore 'ecologies of practice' that promote the development of autonomy are unlikely to develop in a birth centre setting that is overly determined by rigid and codified practices associated with an 'economies of performance' model.

The midwives in the area studied had recently experienced major changes in their work, as well as the closure of their maternity hospital despite their best efforts to retain it. In all of this they can be said to have experienced a loss of autonomy at a political as well as a clinical level. Yet birth centres are associated with considerable autonomy for midwives (Hunter, 2003), and the setting up of such a centre, staffed by midwives from outside the area, must have generated mixed feelings among local midwives, clinicians and managers. Since no help had been available to work through the losses that these midwives had experienced, it is not surprising that their attitude to the Birth Centre and its midwives was less than welcoming.

The Birth Centre midwives had the enthusiasm and knowledge but lacked the authority to undertake tasks that would have strengthened the Birth Centre and increased its bookings (e.g. in publicising the centre, organising a well-publicised opening event or revising its clinical guidelines to include women having their first babies). They did what they could (e.g. by organising the garden parties, with a striking lack of support from midwifery managers), but no one else took on these crucial tasks, and the midwives' frustration mounted.

In the history of this Birth Centre there was no strong, organised user support group that could petition senior management and other professionals. Such a group was crucial to the success of the Edgware Birth Centre (Manero and Turner, 2003), which was set up in otherwise similar circumstances. This is partly because the Birth Centre was instigated by the health authority, not by the local service users. It also shows a lack of strategic vision on the part of the trust, since user involvement was seen as important in the pilot study. However, the Birth Centre was not part of the strategy of the trust. When the numbers of births were growing (between 2002 and 2004), it would have been possible for a strong user group to be created that could have publicised the Birth Centre's presence in the community and argued for its continuance and growth. However, this was just the point at which the service was reduced, the original midwives had left and staff morale had fallen. The community midwives who were then operating the reduced service lacked the authority and the motivation to facilitate a user group.

This Birth Centre was no one's baby, and as such it is scarcely surprising that it failed to thrive.

REFERENCES

Ball L, Curtis P, Kirkham M. *Why Do Midwives Leave?* London: Royal College of Midwives; 2002

Boulton M, Chapple J, Saunders D. Evaluating a new service: clinical outcomes and women's assessments of the Edgware Birth Centre. In: M Kirkham (ed.) *Birth Centres: a social model for maternity care.* Oxford: Books for Midwives; 2003. pp. 115–39.

Brodie P, Leap N. From ideal to real: the interface between birth territory and the maternity services organisation. In: K Fahy, M Fourier, C Hastie (eds) *Birth Territory and Midwifery Guardianship.* Sydney: Books for Midwives; 2008. pp. 149–69.

Davis-Floyd R, Barclay L, Davis B *et al.* (eds). *Birth Models That Work.* Berkeley, CA: University of California Press; 2009.

Deery R. Promoting a sustainable workforce through 'ecologies of practice.' In: L Davies, M Kensington, R Daellenbach (eds) *Sustainability, Midwifery and Birth.* London: Routledge; 2010.

Deery R, Fisher P. 'Switching and swapping' faces: performativity and emotion in midwifery. *International Journal of Work Organisation and Emotion.* 2010; 3: 270–86.

Deery R, Hunter B. Emotion work and relationships in midwifery. In: M Kirkham (ed.) *The Midwife–Mother Relationship*, 2nd edn. Basingstoke: Palgrave Macmillan; 2010.

Fahy K, Fourier M, Hastie C (eds). *Birth Territory and Midwifery Guardianship.* Sydney: Books for Midwives; 2008.

Flint C (ed.) *Communicating Midwifery: twenty years of experience.* Oxford: Books for Midwives; 1995.

Homer C, Brodie P, Leap N (eds). *Midwifery Continuity of Care,* Sydney: Churchill Livingstone; 2008.

Hunter M. Autonomy, clinical freedom and responsibility. In: M Kirkham (ed.) *Birth Centres: a social model for maternity care.* Oxford: Books for Midwives; 2003.

Jones O. Supervision in a midwife-managed birth centre. In: M Kirkham (ed.) *Developments in the Supervision of Midwives.* Manchester: Books for Midwives Press; 2000. pp. 149–68.

Kirkham M. *Basic Supportive Care in Labour.* PhD thesis. Manchester: Faculty of Medicine, University of Manchester; 1987.

Kirkham M (ed.). *Birth Centres: a social model for maternity care.* Oxford: Books for Midwives; 2003.

Manero E, Turner L. Users in the driving seat. In: M Kirkham (ed.) *Birth Centres: a social model for maternity care.* Oxford: Books for Midwives; 2003. pp. 63–70.

Page L (ed.) *The New Midwifery: science and sensitivity in practice.* London: Churchill Livingstone; 2000.

Page L. Being a midwife to midwifery: transforming midwifery services. In: K Fahy,

M Fourier, C Hastie (eds) *Birth Territory and Midwifery Guardianship*. Sydney: Books for Midwives; 2008. pp. 115–29.

Pairman S, Guilliland K. Developing a midwife-led maternity service: the New Zealand experience. In: M Kirkham (ed.) *Birth Centres: a social model for maternity care*. Oxford: Books for Midwives; 2003. pp. 223–38.

Shallow H. The birth centre project. In: M Kirkham (ed.) *Birth Centres: a social model for maternity care*. Oxford: Books for Midwives; 2003. pp. 11–24.

Stronach I, Corbin B, McNamara O *et al*. Towards an uncertain politics of professionalism: teacher and nurse identities in flux. *Journal of Educational Policy*. 2002: **17**: 109–38.

Van der Kooy B. *The NHS Community Midwifery Model*. Abingdon: Independent Midwives UK; 2002. www.onemotheronemidwife.org.uk/The%20NHSCMM.pdf (accessed 10 October 2009).

Walsh D. *Improving Maternity Services: small is beautiful – lessons from a birth centre*. Oxford: Radcliffe Publishing Ltd; 2007.

Walsh D. 'Small really is beautiful': tales from a free-standing birth centre. In: R Davis-Floyd, L Barclay, B Davis *et al*. (eds) *Birth Models That Work*. Berkeley, CA: University of California Press; 2009. pp. 159–86.

CHAPTER 10

Conclusion

Much can be learned from the failure of this Birth Centre to thrive despite the satisfaction of its clients, the quality of the feasibility study, the suitability of the building, and the dedication of the original staff who were specifically appointed to the Birth Centre and many of the community midwives who were subsequently required to work there.

With the planning and moving of full obstetric services away from the town, those who had provided these services experienced real loss. When individuals suffer loss, further change can be experienced as a threat or as the last straw. No help was offered to maternity services staff to deal with this sad situation. This is not a criticism of management in this trust, but a much wider issue for NHS management in an era of centralisation of services.

Three other issues were noted in this research, which have wider relevance. First, no strategic overview for the local maternity services could be discerned from the interviews with managers, or the midwives' reporting of their experience of management. Secondly, there was a lack of transparency with regard to the pressures on the trust. Thus midwives who left were not replaced, and services were reduced without staff having an understanding of why this was happening, which left them feeling powerless. Thirdly, there was no evidence of any strategic efforts to enhance teamworking and improve smooth working between midwives in different work settings and midwives and obstetricians. Such circumstances fostered the continuance of negative coping habits, such as rudeness concerning other groups of staff when clients transfer their care, not consulting staff about proposed changes, or slowness in responding to staff suggestions to improve their service. None of these issues are unique to the trust studied – indeed they are common in NHS maternity services – but they stood in the way of innovation and appeared to stoke a 'fear of excellence' (Page, 1997).

In these circumstances, it was perhaps not surprising that the trust and many of its staff failed to acknowledge that the Birth Centre was offering a social model of care which was very different from the medical model offered in the consultant unit. There were considerable efforts to make the Birth Centre fit with the rest of the trust. Insistence that midwives should wear uniforms, emphasis on what was lacking from a medical viewpoint (e.g. epidurals), and criticism of the centre when inevitably some women required transfer for medical care in labour all demonstrate failure to appreciate the nature of a birth centre. With energetic advocates within the trust, and organised user support, this alternative model could have been explained and publicised, and the dedication of the Birth Centre midwives could have led to the building of a new and special service of which the trust might reasonably be proud. As it was, only one model of care was allowed, and the new model bent to fit and its difference diminished. Thus standardisation can be a sad and limiting other aspect of the centralisation of services.

Standardisation has come to be equated with safety in the management of high-risk births (Practising Midwife, 2009). However, there is a real tension between the desire to craft systems that seek safety through uniform management of patients and the desire of clinicians to craft relationships with individuals in their care (Sennett, 1999). This tension is one of many within modern healthcare that merit public debate, and is especially important in relation to childbirth, where most women are healthy and relationships are all important (Hunter *et al.*, 2008).

This study has shown us much about the circumstances in which a birth centre can fail or thrive. It also raises wider issues of concern which merit public debate, especially concerning contradictions that usually remain masked. These include the need for 'choices for childbearing women and midwives' in reality as well as rhetoric, and acknowledgment of the many factors limiting choice, the need to help people to work together, and the need for strategies to resolve conflict and resistance to change and to increase the self-awareness and personal autonomy of those working around birth. It certainly demonstrates the extent of change which is needed to achieve the choice that is Department of Health policy (Department of Health, 1993, 2004, 2007; Darzi, 2008).

RECOMMENDATIONS

As a result of this research, our extensive reading of the literature on birth centres and our experience of working within these centres, we consider it appropriate to make a number of recommendations that should help those who are considering establishing a birth centre, or who are seeking to retain an existing centre.

1. Birth centres need allies and should have most, and ideally all, of the following:
   - ➤ Support from local service users, preferably a well-organised group that is committed to campaigning for and providing ongoing support for the birth centre.
   - ➤ Midwives who want to work with the autonomy and full use of their skills that a birth centre makes possible. They may not be local, as midwives are willing to relocate for such an opportunity.
   - ➤ Midwifery leadership and management that are committed to the birth centre. This involves leadership within the birth centre with access to senior management and involvement in the forums where the birth centre will be discussed. It also means that there must be at least one senior midwifery manager who is committed to the birth centre and will support it in management forums. These senior managers will facilitate and develop relationships between birth centre staff and those of the obstetric unit with which it is linked and community midwives throughout the locality served by the birth centre. Such managers and leaders would also foster positive relationships between the birth centre and the local community.
   - ➤ Obstetricians in the unit where transfers are received who understand the role of the birth centre.
   - ➤ Supportive GPs (community midwives can achieve much in this regard).
2. Education is important for all involved. Midwives who will be working in a birth centre need training in the skills of normal birth, not just obstetric emergencies. Homebirth midwives are a good source of such skills. Self-awareness and skills of facilitation and relationship are essential for all involved. Learning together can be very helpful. Maternity Service Liaison Committees (MSLCs) often use such training, and may be well placed to give advice. Reflection-on-practice sessions or clinical supervision may be useful and should be designed to meet the needs and develop

the autonomy of those concerned. Role models are all-important. Such education develops more allies for the birth centre.

3. A clear vision and targets for the birth centre need to be agreed and understood by all of the staff who work in or support the birth centre in a service capacity. This means that midwives and doctors who do not work in the birth centre are also encouraged to have a sense of ownership, and to understand how the birth centre is integrated with its obstetric support unit and how it supports the work of that unit. Supportive senior midwifery and medical staff have an important role in restating this ethic and maintaining a shared vision and goals.

4. Public relations are important. The support group can be very helpful here, as can the local press, parish councils, local authorities, MPs and voluntary groups.

5. Regular meetings of all those who support the birth centre can ensure smooth running and be able to anticipate many potential problems.

REFERENCES

Darzi A. *High Quality Care for All*. London: The Stationery Office; 2008.

Department of Health. *Changing Childbirth. Part 1. Report of the Expert Maternity Group*. London: Department of Health; 1993.

Department of Health. *National Service Framework for Children, Young People and Maternity Services*. London: Department of Health; 2004.

Department of Health. *Maternity Matters: choice, access and continuity of care in a safe service*. London: Department of Health; 2007.

Hunter B, Berg M, Lundgren I *et al.* Relationships: the hidden threads in the tapestry of maternity care. *Midwifery*. 2008; 24: 132–7.

Page L. Misplaced values: in fear of excellence. *British Journal of Midwifery*. 1997; **5**: 652–4.

Practising Midwife. Computer systems could manage high-risk births. *Practising Midwife*. 2009; **12**: 8.

Sennett R. *The Corrosion of Character: The personal consequences of work in the New Capitalism*. London: WW Norton & Company; 1999.

Index